SELF-ASSESSMENT F

Clinical Medicine

Charles D Forbes DSc, MD, FRCP, FRSE
Professor of Medicine
Ninewells Hospital and Medical School
Dundee, Scotland

William F Jackson MA, MB, BChir, MRCP
formerly Honorary Consultant
Department of Medicine
Guy's Hospital, London

and

Christopher Thompson MD, MRCP
Senior Registrar
Department of Medicine
Ninewells Hospital and Medical School
Dundee, Scotland

ᛞ Mosby-Wolfe

London Baltimore Bogotá Boston Buenos Aires Caracas Carlsbad, CA Chicago Madrid Mexico City Milan Naples, FL
New York Philadelphia St. Louis Sydney Tokyo Toronto Wiesbaden

Copyright © 1995 Times Mirror International Publishers Limited

Published in 1995 by Mosby-Wolfe, an imprint of Times Mirror International Publishers Limited

Project Manager Roderick Craig

Acquisition Editor Claire Hooper

Publisher Geoff Greenwood

Production Controller Mike Heath

Printed in Spain by Grafos, S.A. ARTE SOBRE PAPEL

ISBN 0 723 42118 8

All rights reserved. No part of this publication may be reproduced, stored in a retrieval system, copied or transmitted, in any form or by any means, electronic, mechanical, photocopying, recording or otherwise without written permission from the Publisher or in accordance with the provisions of the Copyright Act 1956 (as amended), or under the terms of any licence permitting limited copying issued by the Copyright Licensing Agency, 33–34 Alfred Place, London, WC1E 7DP.

Any person who does any unauthorised act in relation to this publication may be liable to criminal prosecution and civil claims for damages.

Permission to photocopy or reproduce solely for internal or personal use is permitted for libraries or other users registered with the Copyright Clearance Center, provided that the base fee of $4.00 per chapter plus $.10 per page is paid directly to the Copyright Clearance Center, 21 Congress Street, Salem, MA 01970. This consent does not extend to other kinds of copying, such as copying for general distribution, for advertising or promotional purposes, for creating new collected works, or for resale.

For full details of all Times Mirror International Publishers Limited titles, please write to Times Mirror International Publishers Limited, Lynton House, 7–12 Tavistock Square, London WC1H 9LB, England.

A CIP catalogue record for this book is available from the British Library.

Library of Congress Cataloging-in-Publication Data applied for.

PREFACE

This book is intended as a visual revision aid for those working for the MRCP examination and equivalent examinations in the rest of the world, and as an enjoyable tool for undergraduate and post-graduate students of medicine at all stages. Its range is similar to that of *A Colour Atlas and Text of Clinical Medicine* (Forbes & Jackson; Mosby-Wolfe 1993) and we hope that it will make a useful companion to that volume. Further information on most of the conditions appearing here can be found there, but this book can, of course, be used alone or with reference to other textbooks.

ACKNOWLEDGEMENTS

All the illustrations in this book are, to the best of our knowledge, published here for the first time. Approximately 150 of them came from our own collections, while the rest were lent to us by a number of colleagues, including Dr Ray Newton, Dr Danny Sinclair, Dr Stuart Pringle, Pat Lomax, Dr Leslie Jackson, Dr John Winter, Dr Harry Gray, Professor Martin Pippard, Dr Jill Belch, Dr Norman Kennedy, Dr Michael James, Dr Chris Pennington, Dr Rona McMenamin, Dr Graeme McNeil, Dr Graham Lowe, Dr John Baillie and Professor Alfred Cuschieri. We would like to thank them and also the medical photographers who took many of the pictures.

Charles Forbes
William Jackson
Christopher Thompson

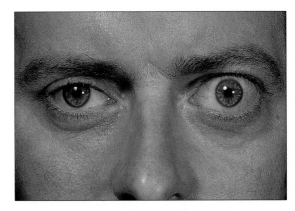

1. This 40-year-old man presented to the medical clinic with a history of two months' progressive weight loss. What abnormality is shown and what is the differential diagnosis?

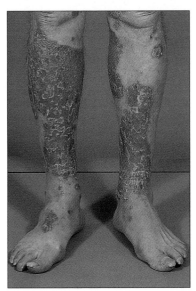

2. Describe this condition and its appropriate treatment.

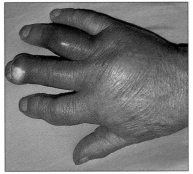

3. This 57-year-old man developed these acute changes in his right hand after starting a course of frusemide to treat his congestive cardiac failure. What are the three main abnormalities shown? How should he be treated for this?

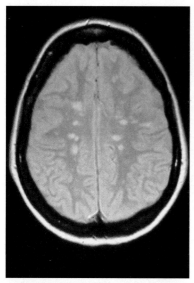

4. What technique has been used to produce this picture? What is the major abnormality and what is the underlying diagnosis?

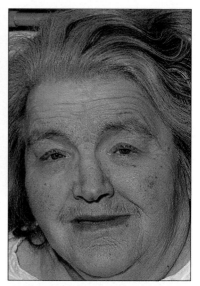

5. This 60-year-old patient was seen at the clinic because of severe angina of effort. What background disease is suggested by her facial appearance, what other features are likely to be present and how should she be managed?

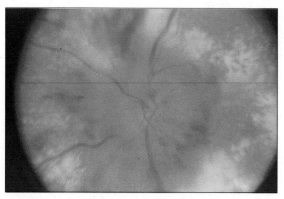

6. This 43-year-old patient presented with recent-onset severe frontal headache. Examination of the fundi revealed the appearance shown. Describe the changes and suggest what acute treatment is needed.

7. What is this common abnormality called and from what does it result?

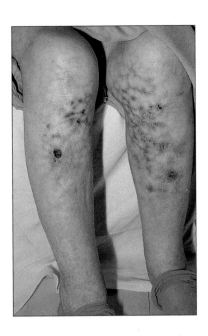

8. This 59-year-old man presented with a painful, swollen right arm, the symptoms of which started at the end of a golfing holiday in which he was playing 36 holes per day. Prior to this he had never been unwell. What is the diagnosis, how should it be investigated and what is the treatment?

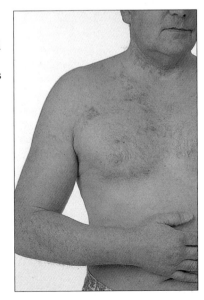

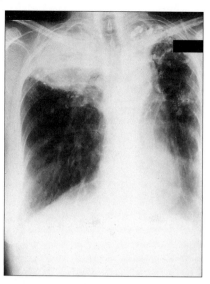

9. This patient, a 55-year-old man, presented with haemoptysis. He had two conditions, one of which is a long-term complication of the other. What are they?

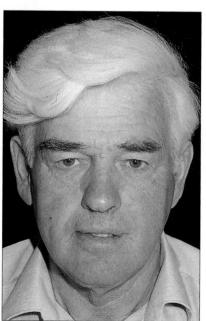

10. This man was referred to the haematology clinic because of symptoms of progressive anaemia. This picture was taken on referral, when he was 45 years old, but his hair had been white for the past 20 years. What is the most likely diagnosis, and what are the characteristics of this form of the anaemia?

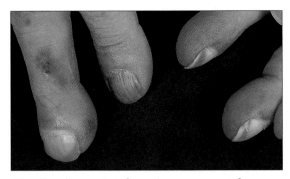

11. What diagnostic information can you get from examination of these fingers? What underlying abnormalities may be associated with the major feature?

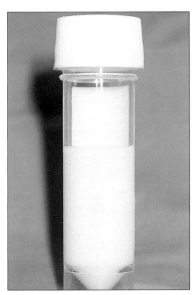

12. This fluid was obtained as a pleural aspirate. What is it called and what has caused the appearance?

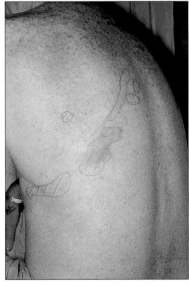

13. This is a 55-year-old seaman who presented with itchy lesions on his flank and back. These have been outlined in ink to show them better. What is the condition called and what are the causes?

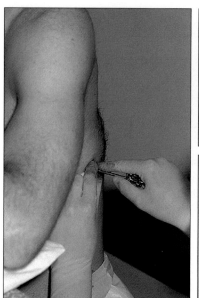
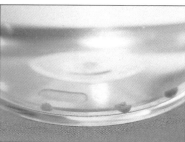
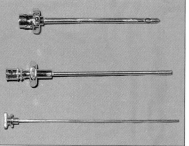

14. What procedure is being carried out here and how is it performed? What is the name of the instrument? The top right picture shows the end result of the procedure and the lower right picture shows the components of the instrument.

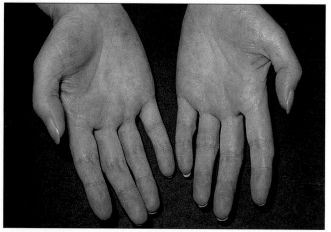

15. What is this appearance called and what is its significance?

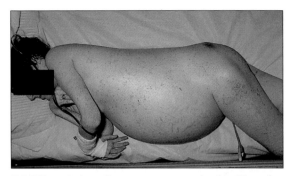

16. What obvious features are present in this 38-year-old comatose woman?

17. This 46-year-old man was admitted with acute myocardial infarction, as confirmed by serial enzyme elevation (CK-MB) and acute changes in his electrocardiogram. Routine examination showed these abnormalities in his hands. What are they and what are the implications?

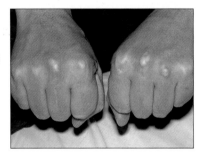

18. This patient presented at the vascular clinic with severe Raynaud's phenomenon and ischaemic ulceration of the tips of her fingers. Describe the abnormalities in her facial appearance. What is the diagnosis and what other symptoms and signs may she have?

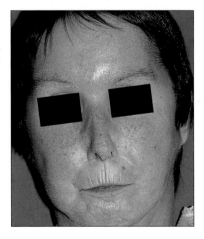

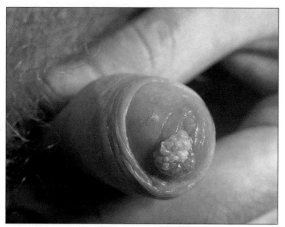

19. This 37-year-old man presented at a sexually transmitted disease clinic, fearing that he had contracted a venereal infection. Several of his close friends had developed severe perianal warts and he thought that he might have developed this condition also following anal intercourse. What is the lesion shown and how should it be investigated?

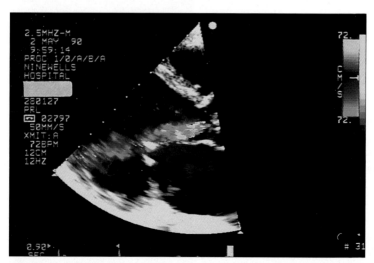

20. What technique has been used here and what abnormality is shown?

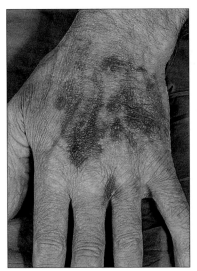

21. What is the abnormality in this 78-year-old woman and what is it due to? Similar changes were widespread over her hands and forearms.

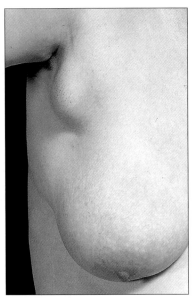

22. Describe the obvious abnormality in this patient.

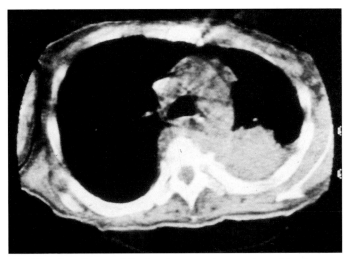

23. What imaging modality has been used to produce this picture and what does it show?

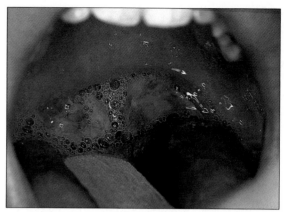

24. This 18-year-old male complained of a sore throat accompanied by difficulty in swallowing. The symptoms had been present for two days. He also felt generally unwell and thought he might have had a slight pyrexia for the past week. What abnormalities are shown in the throat and what are the possible causes?

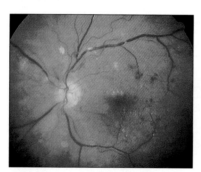

25. Describe the changes shown in this picture of the optic fundus. What is the probable diagnosis?

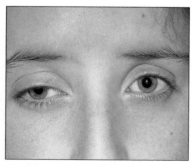

26. This girl was seen with diplopia, which was of sudden onset. What are the abnormalities on inspection of the eyes, seen here as the patient looks at the camera?

27. These painful lesions developed on the thighs and shins of a 22-year-old man. What is the diagnosis and what are the common causes? Where else may the lesions be seen?

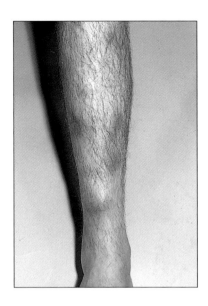

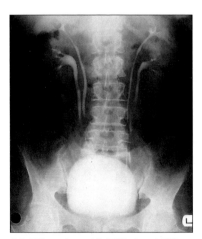

28. What does this IVP show? What is the significance of this abnormality?

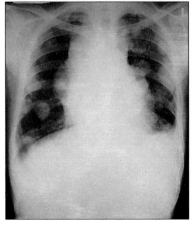

29. This 62-year-old man was admitted with weight loss and progressive dyspnoea on exertion. What abnormalities are shown in the x-ray of his chest? What are the likely causes?

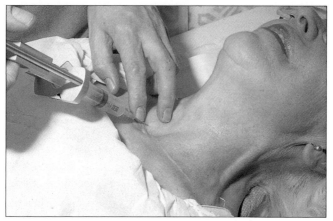

30. What procedure is being carried out here and when is it required?

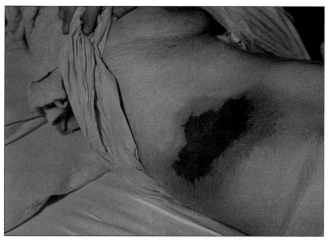

31. This lady had elective surgery for a hip replacement seven days prior to this picture being taken. She subsequently developed a deep-vein thrombosis in her left calf and thigh. Two days before the picture was taken, therapy with heparin and warfarin was started. On the day of the photograph, a lesion had also developed acutely in her right flank, as shown. What is it and what is the mechanism?

32. This 56-year-old male had a laparotomy for a mass lesion in the caecum. This was shown histologically to be a carcinoma of the colon and he underwent a right hemicolectomy four days prior to this picture being taken. What is the complication and how should it be treated?

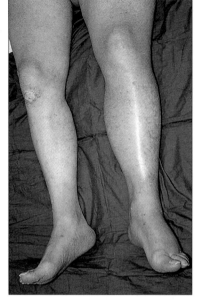

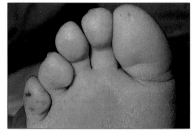

33. A known 17-year-old drug addict was admitted with pain and swelling of the right inguinal region. It was thought that she had an abscess in her groin. What features are present in her foot and what is causing them?

34. What abnormality in the gums is shown here and what is its commonest cause?

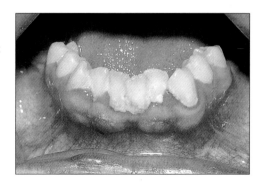

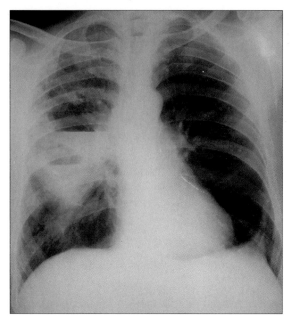

35. This patient spent the night in a police cell after being found drunk and disorderly. He was discharged the following morning, but was later admitted to hospital with pneumonia. What are the appearances on the *x*-ray?

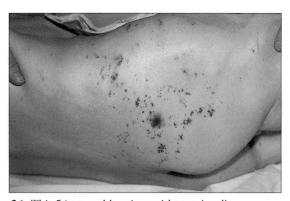

36. This 56-year-old patient with non-insulin dependent diabetes developed a large boil on his thigh and became severely ill. He was in diabetic ketoacidosis when admitted, with this appearance on the skin of his buttocks and a temperature of 39.8° (102°F). What is the cause, and what investigations are required?

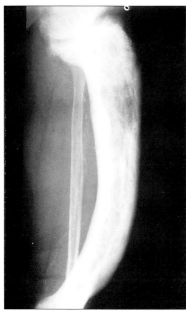

37. What abnormalities are shown in this *x*-ray of the tibia and what is the diagnosis?

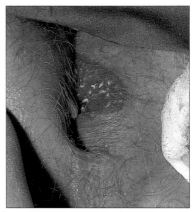

38. This patient, who was being followed up in the long-term after the successful treatment of thyrotoxicosis, complained that he had been bothered by "piles" for the past six months. He had applied a variety of local agents but that they had got worse and were now bleeding. What is shown in this picture?

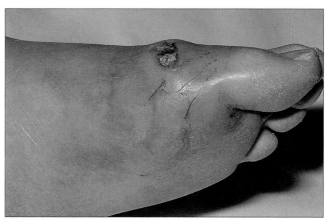

39. What lesion is shown here on the foot? What is the most likely underlying disorder?

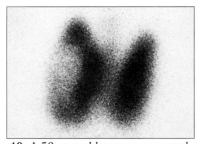

40. A 58-year-old woman presented with a swelling in her neck. What test has been done and what does it show?

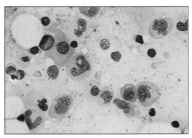

41. This patient presented with severe anaemia. What are the appearances in the bone marrow? The patient had prematurely grey hair. What is the likely diagnosis?

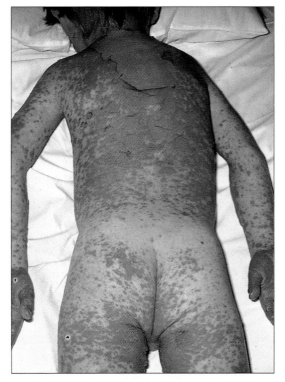

42. What is the diagnosis in this acutely ill child and what is the usual cause?

43. What are the lesions on the lips and what is their treatment?

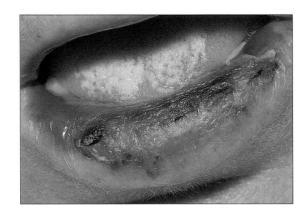

44. Describe the main abnormalities in this woman's face. What is the likely cause and how may the condition be treated?

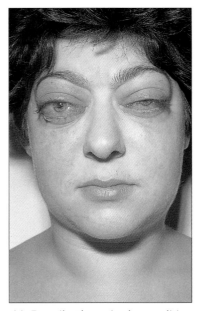

45. This man has long-standing weakness of grip in the left hand. What two abnormalities are present?

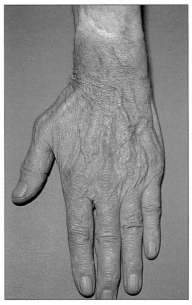

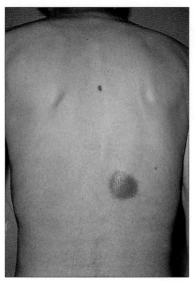

46. This patient had been generally unwell for several weeks, with occasional low-grade fever, some weight loss, extreme fatigue and anorexia. His wife drew attention to this lesion on his back, which seemed to be rapidly increasing in size. What are the clinical possibilities and how may the diagnosis be reached?

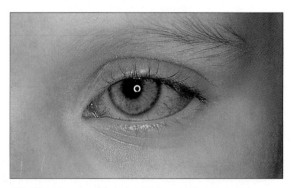

47. This 6-year-old male child was admitted with a history of two days' acute onset of fever, ulcerative gingivitis and rhinitis, associated with pronounced enlargement of cervical lymph nodes on both sides of the neck. In addition there was a history of some general discomfort in the small joints of both hands and feet. What additional clinical sign is shown in this picture and how could this disorder lead to serious cardiovascular problems?

48. This 56-year-old woman was seen in the casualty department after passing fresh red blood per rectum on defaecation. There was a history extending over two years of recurrent, niggling left iliac fossa pain and she had had episodes of diarrhoea, often associated with left-sided lower abdominal pain. What kind of *x*-ray is this and what does it show? What further investigation is indicated? How should she be treated?

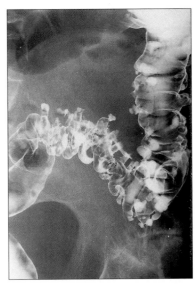

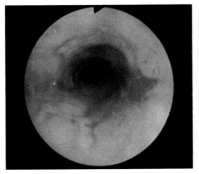 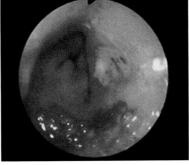

49. This 56-year-old female underwent upper gastrointestinal endoscopy for recurrent dyspepsia. What two abnormalities are present in the mid-oesophagus (above left) and the lower oesophagus (above right).

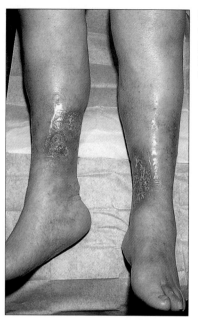

50. This woman was sent for an opinion concerning the long-standing problem with her legs. What signs are present in this picture and what is causing them?

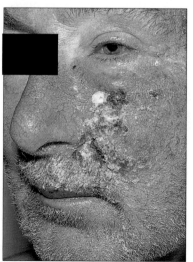

51. Eight days before this picture was taken the patient had complained of a tingling pain starting in his left cheek. This was rapidly followed by the appearance of multiple vesicles that burst, leaving an erythematous base. The lesions mainly affected the cheek and extended to the mid-line. They they were also present in the buccal mucosa. What is the disease and what potential complications may it have?

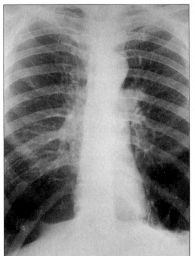
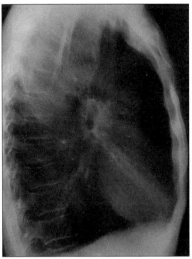

52. This 59-year-old man was referred with progressive dyspnoea at rest. What is the diagnosis and what features are shown in these x-rays of his chest?

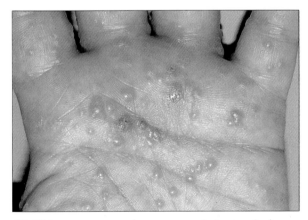

53. This young woman has recurrent, irritant vesicular lesions on her hands. She has also had atopic eczema from early childhood onwards, although this is now a relatively minor problem. What is the diagnosis, and what are the possible provoking factors of her condition?

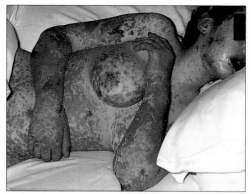

54. This 27-year-old woman was admitted severely ill with fever, bilateral conjunctivitis, extensive inflammation of the mucosa of the mouth and genital tract and a widespread rash with desquamation over her entire body. What is this condition? What causes it and how is the patient managed?

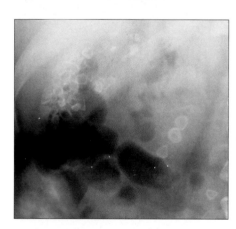

55. This 47-year-old woman was admitted as an emergency with nausea, vomiting and acute, colicky type pain in the right upper quadrant. A plain *x*-ray of the abdomen is shown. Describe the abnormality. What is the management of such a patient?

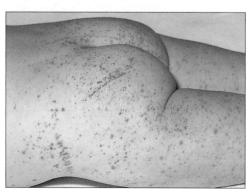

56. This 7-year-old boy presented to the out-patient clinic with a one-day history of low-grade fever, diffuse upper alimentary pain, discomfort in both knees and the appearances in this picture. What features are shown and what is the disease?

57. This 60-year-old man was being treated for a pneumonia that was slow to resolve. He developed these vesicular eruptions in several areas of his skin. What was the probable causative organism of his pneumonia and what other complications should be looked for?

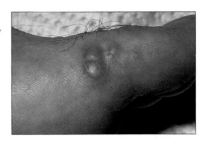

58. This 56-year-old woman presented acutely with abrupt onset of fever, rigors, headache and swelling around the left eye. What is shown here? What are the common causes of the problem and how is it treated?

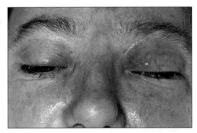

59. This 23-year-old male had been receiving treatment at a follow-up clinic with a diagnosis of ulcerative colitis, which had recently flared up. He came complaining of the sudden appearance of some lesions on his skin, which had been present for the past week. What is this complication and how should it be managed? What other conditions may be associated with it?

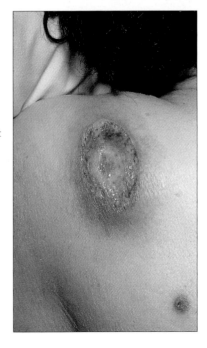

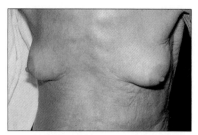

60. This 72-year-old man has been receiving treatment for the past six months for carcinoma of the prostate. What caused the complication shown here? What other disorders and drugs may cause the same problem?

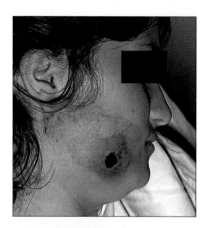

61. This lesion developed slowly and progressively over several weeks; it seemed to be related to dental extraction three months earlier, which had been carried out because of an underlying dental abscess. What is the cause of the lesion and how should it be treated?

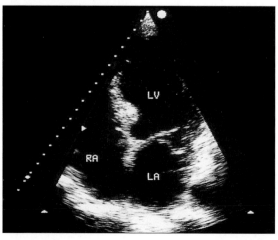

62. This test was carried out on a fit 27-year-old woman who presented with an episode of acute dyspnoea that resolved rapidly with rest. What test has been done and what does it show?

63. What abnormalities are shown in this patient's facies? What is the most likely diagnosis? How does the pale patch on the bridge of the nose relate to the other findings?

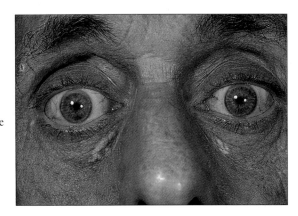

64. What obvious lesion is shown in this girl? What are the likely causes in females of this age?

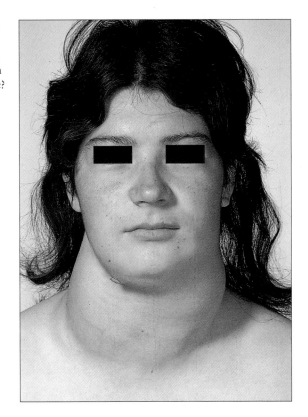

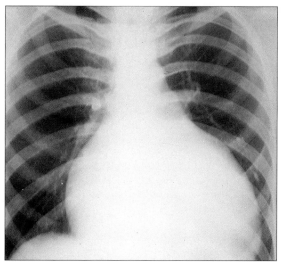

65. This is a PA chest *x*-ray of a patient admitted with a history of chest pain one week prior to this episode. What does it show?

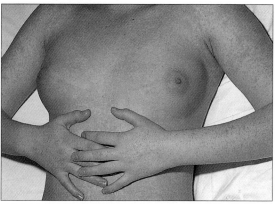

66. This 17-year-old girl had been unwell for several days with a mild fever and sore throat. She also developed tender, enlarged cervical lymph nodes. What is the likely diagnosis? What important additional questions should be asked?

67. This 22-year-old man had been ill for at least ten days before presentation. There was a history of irritation and redness of the eyes, and swelling of both knee joints. What is this genital lesion, and what is the underlying diagnosis? What factor may predispose men to this disorder?

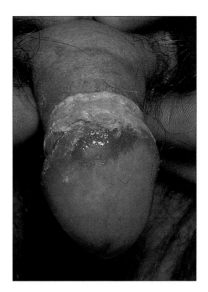

68. This 55-year-old male had presented with haematemesis. What type of x-ray has been done and what is the pathology shown?

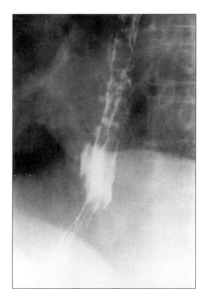

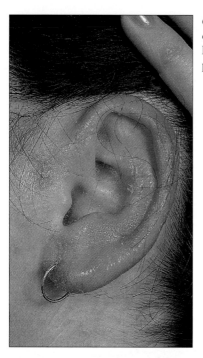

69. This girl came to the surgery complaining of itchiness and weeping lesions on her ear. What disorder is present and what is the likely cause?

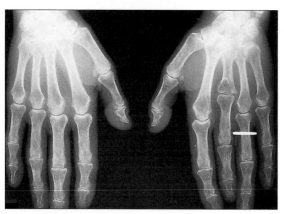

70. What is the obvious abnormality in this *x*-ray of a patient's hands.

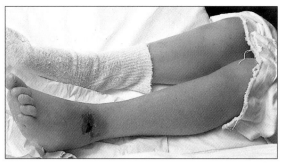

71. This patient presented with a painful, swollen calf and was undergoing appropriate investigations. What medically induced complication has developed?

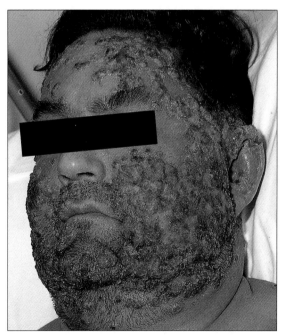

72. This man had a systemic illness with high fever and cervical lymphadenopathy. What is the diagnosis and the cause of the man's rash?

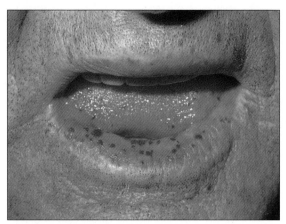

73. This patient has a history of chronic anaemia.
What is the diagnosis? What management is required?

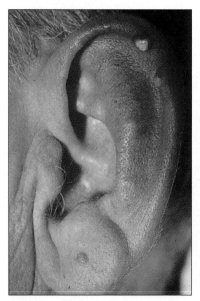

74. What is the lesion on this man's
ear?

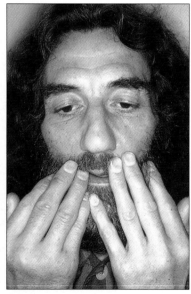

75. This 37-year-old man had a
long history of tiredness and lethargy.
What is the obvious problem?

76. What is the cause of the abnormality of this man's tongue?

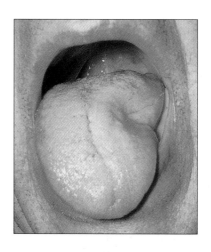

77. This is the neck of a 67-year-old woman, who is sitting up in bed. What abnormality is shown and how should its significance be assessed?

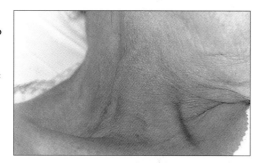

78. This is the lateral view of the abdomen of a 74-year-old man. What abnormality is present?

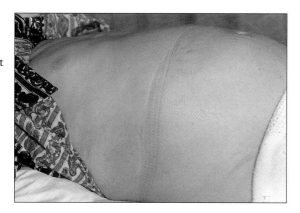

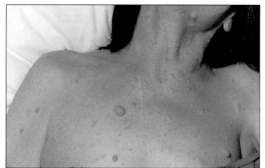

79. This 58-year-old woman was found on routine screening to have hypertension of an intermittent type and an underlying chronic disorder. What is the abnormality shown and what is its association with hypertension?

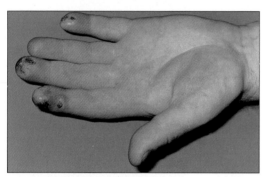

80. This 45-year-old man has a condition which is more commonly seen in women. What abnormalities are shown on the hand, and what is the underlying diagnosis?

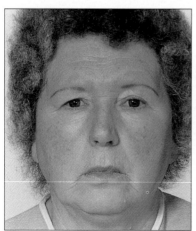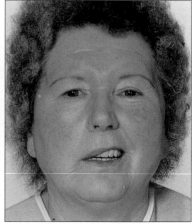

81. This lady has been asked to smile. What lesion is demonstrated?

82. This 24-year-old boy had been suffering from ulcerative colitis for four years. He had been treated with steroid enemas, courses of systemic steroids and sulphasalazine. He presented acutely with a swollen tender abdomen. What abnormality is shown and how should it be treated?

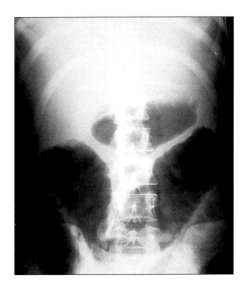

83. This sexually active young man presented at the genito-urinary medicine clinic. What are the lesions and what is their cause and treatment?

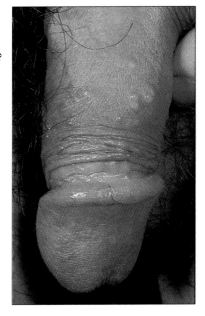

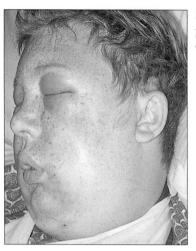

84. Describe the changes in this patient's facies. What is the likely diagnosis and what are its major causes?

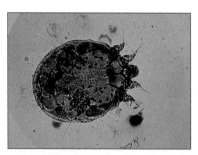

85. This image was produced from material removed from a skin lesion on the back of a patient's hand, near the inter-digital cleft. What does it show?

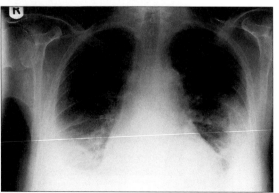

86. What abnormalities are shown in this PA *x*-ray of the chest of a 54-year-old man.

87. This 32-year-old woman presented with infertility, but she gave a long history of abdominal distension and diarrhoea, for which she had received only symptomatic treatment. What abnormalities are shown and what is the likely underlying cause? How should the patient be managed?

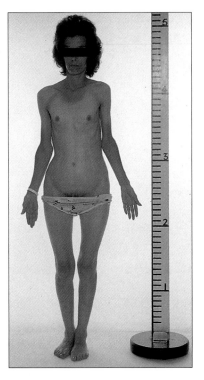

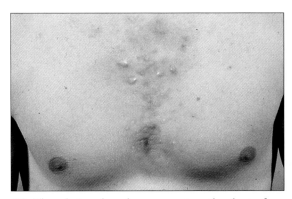

88. These lesions have been present on the chest of this 19-year-old man for the past 2 years. What is the likely diagnosis?

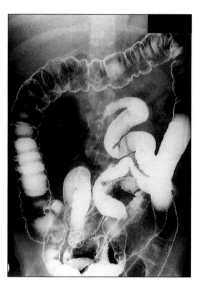

89. What kind of procedure has been carried out here and what does it show?

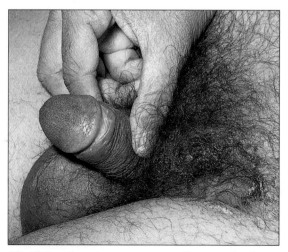

90. This patient was seen at a sexually transmitted disease clinic. His inguinal lymph nodes were enlarged. What abnormalities are demonstrated here and what is their likely cause?

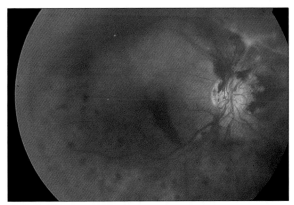

91. Describe the abnormalities seen in the retina of this patient. What is the likely cause?

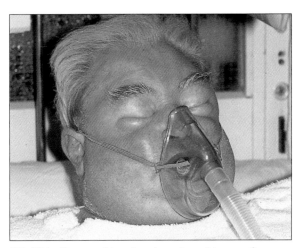

92. This 61-year-old patient has a long history of chronic obstructive airways disease. On this occasion he was admitted with sudden onset of chest pain following a prolonged bout of coughing. X-ray of the chest confirmed the presence of a tension pneumothorax on the left. An intrapleural catheter was inserted and attached to an underwater seal drain, but he suddenly deteriorated, with extreme swelling of the face and neck. What complication has occurred?

41

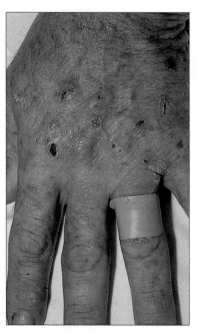

93. This patient has an inherited metabolic disorder. Describe the changes in the hand and suggest a diagnosis.

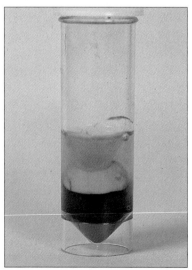

94. This blood sample was taken for serology and allowed to stand for 20 minutes. What is shown here?

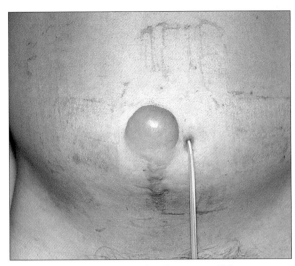

95. This middle-aged man has been unwell for some time, with insidious development of renal failure. What procedure has been carried out and what complication has resulted?

96. This 48-year-old Caucasian man was sent to the diabetes clinic for investigation of hyperglycaemia. His fasting blood sugar confirmed that he was frankly diabetic. What additional diagnosis should be considered on examination of his facies?

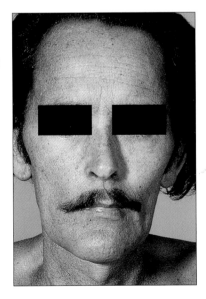

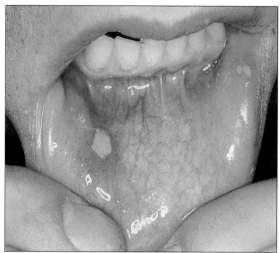

97. What is the condition shown here and with what diseases may it be associated?

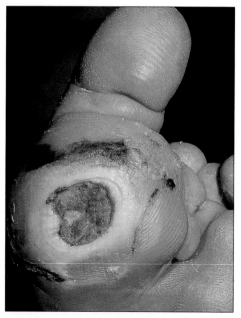

98. Describe the abnormalities seen here. What is the likely diagnosis?

99. This 70-year-old man presented with sudden loss of vision in the right eye. What is the likely diagnosis, what other symptoms may have preceded the blindness and how would you confirm the diagnosis?

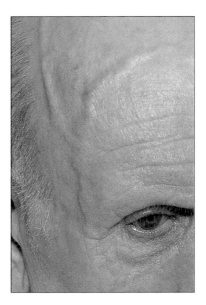

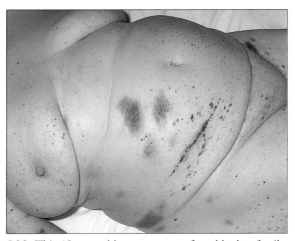

100. This 49-year-old woman was referred by her family doctor because of severe and persisting ulcerating tonsillitis and pharyngitis. What features are now manifesting in her skin, what is the likely diagnosis and what are the common causes of this condition?

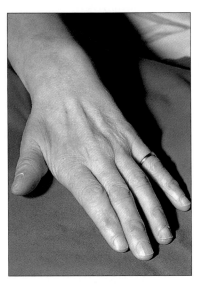

101. This is the hand of a 46-year-old man; there are no sensory abnormalities. Describe the appearances. What is the likely diagnosis?

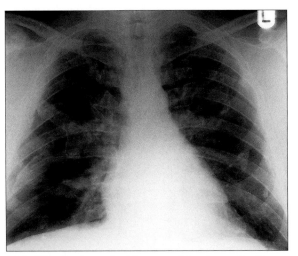

102. What is shown in this x-ray of the chest of a 65-year-old retired shipyard worker? What is the cause of the abnormalities? How is his smoking history relevant?

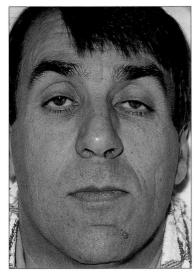 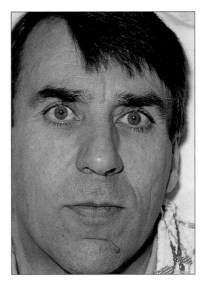

103. What sign is shown above left? What has happened prior to the picture above right, taken 5 minutes later? What is the diagnosis?

104. What are the obviously abnormal clinical signs in this 48-year-old woman? What is the likely diagnosis?

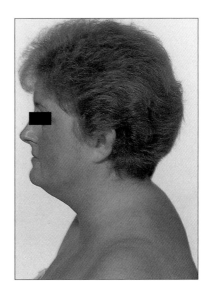

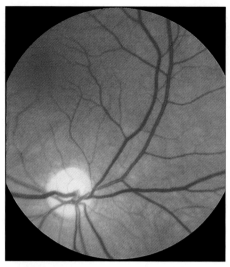

105. This is the fundal photograph of a patient with acromegaly. What does it show and what is the explanation for this finding?

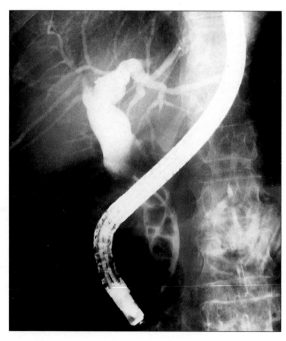

106. What is this investigation and what does it show? Give three ways in which the patient might present.

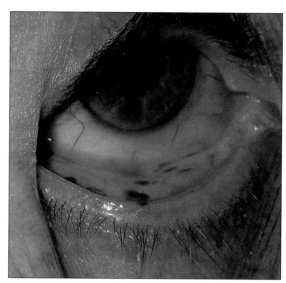

107. This 58-year-old man presented with left upper quadrant abdominal pain four weeks after dental extraction. What physical signs are shown in the picture? What is the probable diagnosis and what is the cause of the abdominal pain?

108. What does this radiograph show and what is the likely underlying diagnosis?

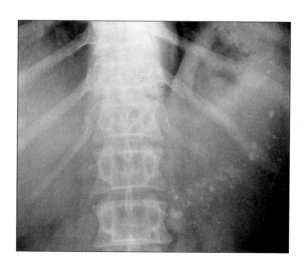

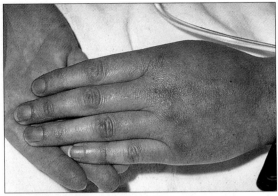

109. This 28-year-old man with small bowel disease was prescribed a special diet and medication for a skin rash. There was no evidence of cardiac or respiratory disease. What is the cause of the appearance of his hand (compared here with a normal hand), what drug is he receiving, what is his skin rash and what is the nature of his small bowel disease?

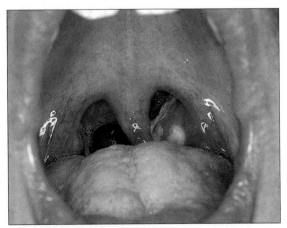

110. A 17-year-old boy presented with fever, pain radiating to the left ear on swallowing and this appearance in the oral cavity. What is the diagnosis, what is the likely pathogen and what treatment is indicated?

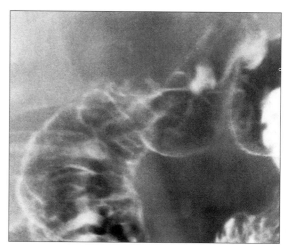

111. This patient has a long history of epigastric pain. What kind of x-ray examination has been carried out and what does it show? What further investigation is indicated?

112. This 63-year-old man presented acutely with fever, pain and swelling of his penis and scrotum. What is the diagnosis?

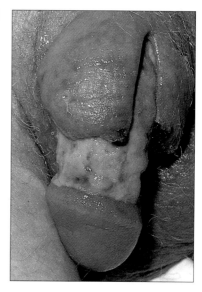

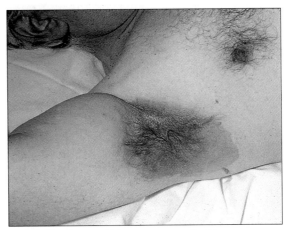

113. This 71-year-old man presented with nausea, weight loss and an iron-deficiency anaemia. Physical examination revealed this skin appearance. What is the lesion and the most likely underlying diagnosis?

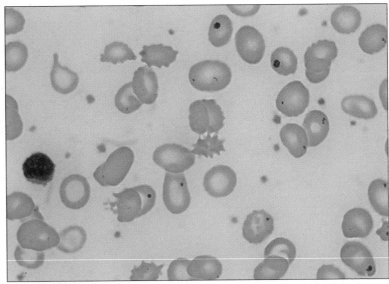

114. What changes are present in this blood film? What special risk is the patient subject to?

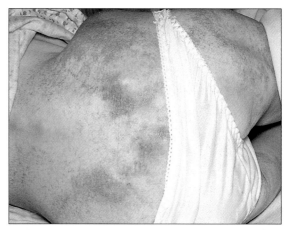

115. This 24-year-old woman with severe Crohn's disease is receiving parenteral nutrition. Describe the physical signs. What is the likely cause of the rash? What other symptoms may be present?

116. This 52-year-old Caucasian woman presented with lassitude, weight loss and hypotension. What is the probable diagnosis and how would you confirm it?

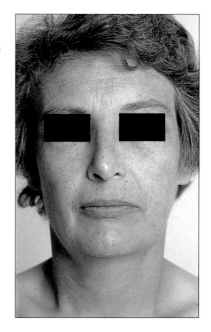

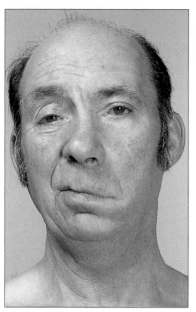

117. Describe the abnormalities on the face of this 68-year-old man who has been asked to smile. What is the diagnosis and the prognosis?

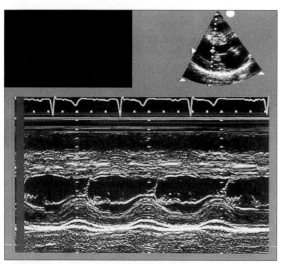

118. What kind of tracing is this and what is the probable diagnosis?

119. The 9am serum cortisol of this 16-year-old boy was not suppressed during an overnight dexamethasone suppression test, but he showed a normal serum cortisol response to insulin-induced hypoglycaemia. What two physical signs are present and what is the diagnosis?

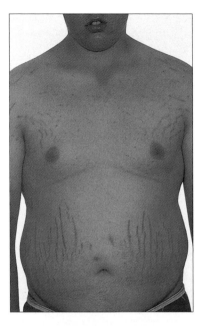

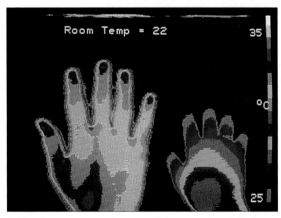

120. These are two pictures of the same hand, before (left) and after (right) a test. What type of test has been carried out, and what is the imaging technique? What is the cause of the changes and what is the diagnosis?

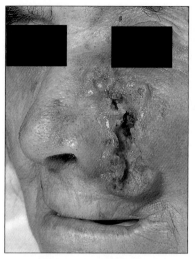

121. This elderly man had been reclusive since the death of his wife three years prior to his admission. He was admitted one winter's night after his neighbours had not seen any signs of life at his house for some days. He was suffering from extreme neglect and hypothermia. What is the lesion on his face and how should it be treated?

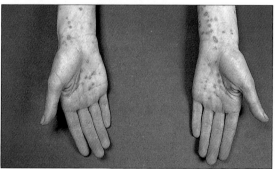

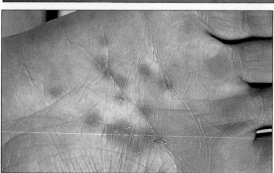

122. This 19-year-old girl had been living in a commune for the past year, during which time she had developed a drug habit. She presented with this rash, which was generalized over her entire body, including the palms of her hands and soles of her feet. What are the possible causes?

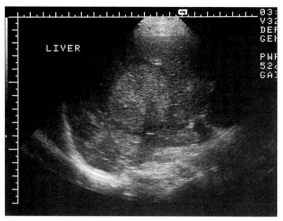

123. What kind of investigation is shown here and what abnormalities are present?

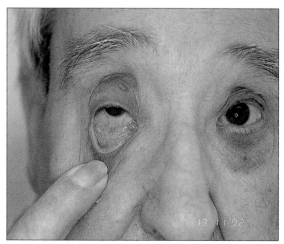

124. List three abnormalities seen on examination of this man's facies.

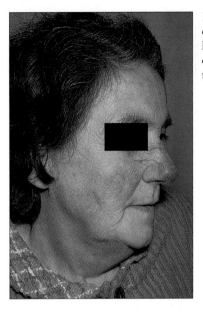

125. This patient has a multisystem disorder. What lesion is present on her face? What is the underlying disorder? With what other disorders can the facial abnormality be confused?

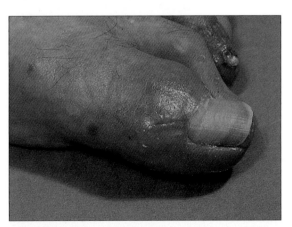

126. This patient was known to have long-standing, extensive psoriasis that had been treated intermittently over many years. He now gave a history of a recent discharge of white material from the toes. What is the likely cause, and how is it associated with the underlying psoriasis?

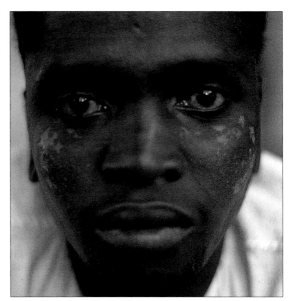

127. This patient presented to the rheumatology clinic with polyarthritis. Describe the facial lesion. What is the probable underlying diagnosis?

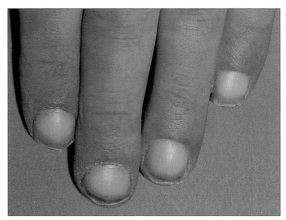

128. Describe the appearances of the nails. What are the common causes of this condition?

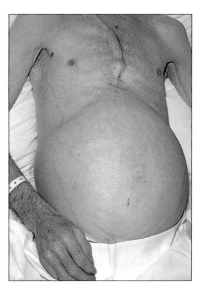

137. What abnormalities are present in this 58-year-old man?

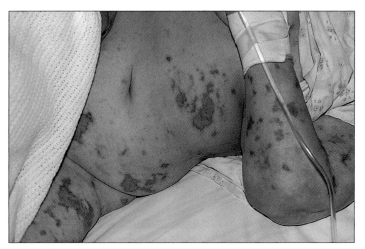

138. This patient was admitted as an emergency. He had been seen 40 minutes previously by his family doctor and admission was arranged because of his high swinging fever and rigors. The abnormality shown here developed during this 40-minute period. What is its cause and what emergency treatment is required to save the man's life?

139. What is shown in this specimen pot and what is the colour due to?

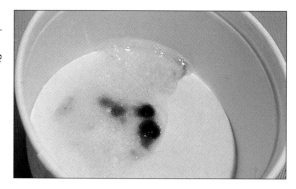

140. What two abnormalities are shown in this x-ray of the chest of a 67-year-old man.

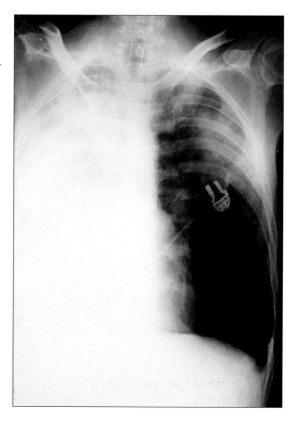

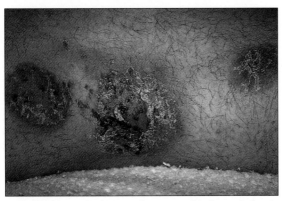

141. What are the lesions shown on this farmer's legs? They were intensely itchy. How would you confirm the diagnosis?

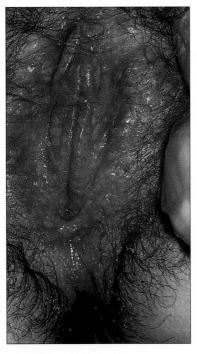

142. This 24-year-old medical student had been on holiday in Greece. On her return she was obviously ill with pyrexia, extreme local discomfort in the perineum and pain on micturition. There was no local vaginal discharge. What is the likely diagnosis?

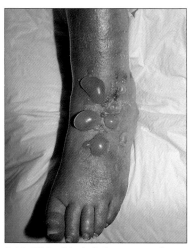

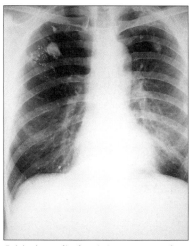

143. This elderly lady presented with a recurrence of a previously diagnosed blistering disease. What is the diagnosis? At what level in the skin do the blisters form?

144. A medical opinion was sought as a result of this routine pre-surgery x-ray of a patient's chest. What does it show? Is this a cause for concern?

145. This 65-year-old man has been unwell for the past month with the gradual onset of weakness, particularly of the pelvic girdle muscles but also affecting his shoulder. He also complained of some muscle discomfort. These features were particularly noticeable when he tried to get out of a low armchair or climb stairs. He had also been aware of a red skin rash over his face. What is the likely diagnosis and what additional laboratory tests may be of value?

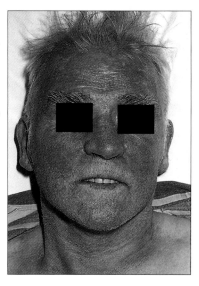

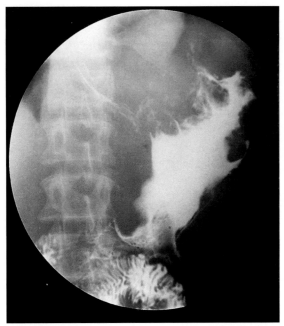

146. What kind of x-ray is this and what does it show?

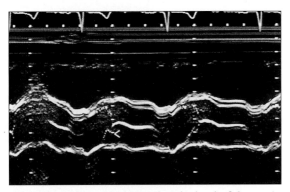

147. This image was obtained at the level of the aortic root. What is it and what does it show?

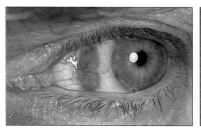 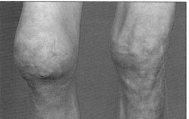

148. What abnormality is shown in this patient's eye? How is it linked to the abnormality in his knees?

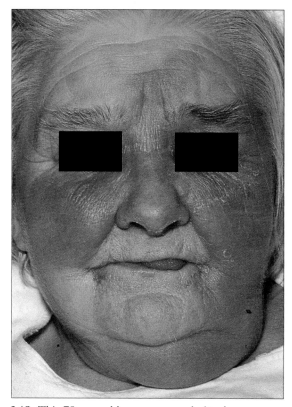

149. This 78-year-old woman was admitted as an emergency with high fever and rigors. What abnormality is shown in her face? What is its cause?

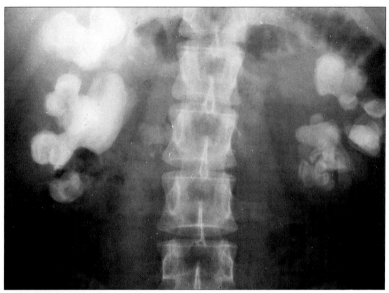

150. What is shown in this plain x-ray of the abdomen?

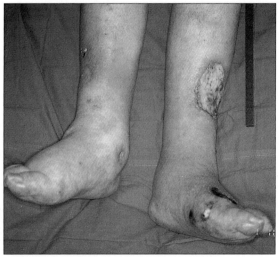

151. What is shown in this picture and what is the background disease?

152. The lesion on the face of this 52-year-old man presented originally as a subcutaneous nodule that enlarged rapidly over the following two months. What are the possible diagnoses?

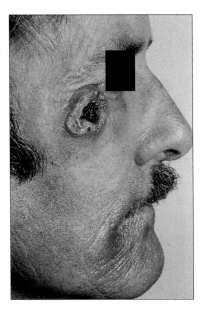

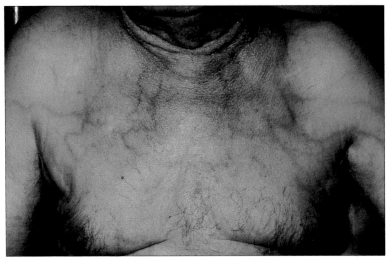

153. This picture was taken in infra-red light. What abnormal features are shown and what is their cause?

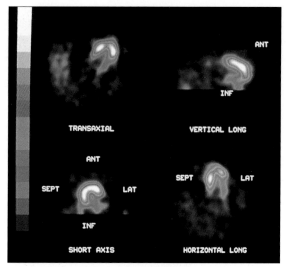

154. How are these images of the heart at peak exercise produced and what do they show?

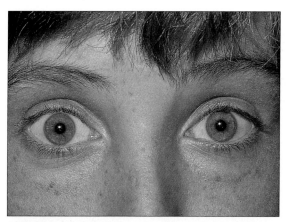

155. This 15-year-old boy has been suffering from this nephrotic syndrome for some years, despite the use of steroid therapy. He continues to have marked proteinuria but his generalized oedema has settled. What long term complication of the disease is suggested by the appearance of his eyes?

156. What are the lesions shown here?

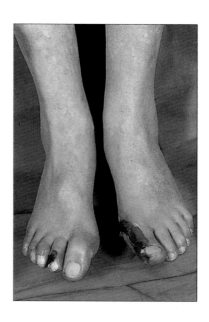

157. What abnormalities are shown in this 42-year-old man?

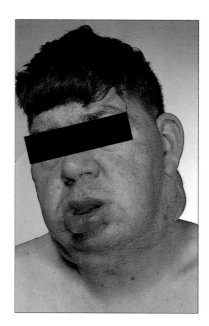

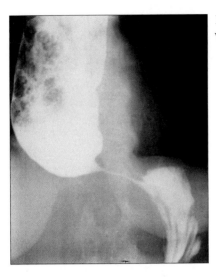

158. What kind of *x*-ray is this and what pathology does it reveal?

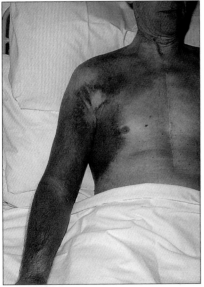

159. This 53-year-old man had a knee joint replacement that was complicated by the development of a deep-vein thrombosis, despite the use of prophylactic low-dose heparin. He was treated initially with therapeutic heparin and warfarin and discharged with a stable INR of 2.9 on a dose of 6mg warfarin/day. Four days after this he presented with the appearances shown. What has happened and what is the most likely cause?

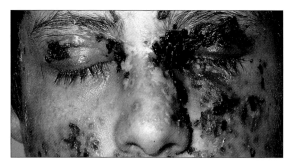

160. This patient, who was known to suffer from eczema, developed this severe eruption. What is the cause and how is it treated?

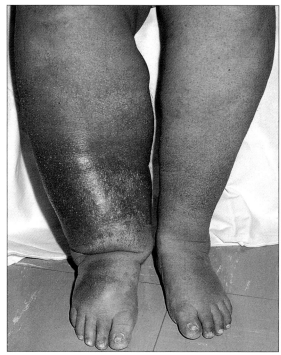

161. This woman has a fever and general malaise. What acute disease has supervened on a long-standing problem?

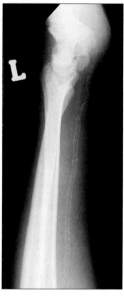

162. What abnormality is shown in this *x*-ray of the arm?

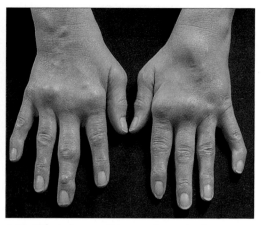

163. What abnormalities are shown in these hands? What is the likely diagnosis?

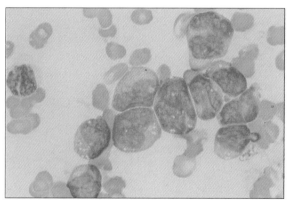

164. What diagnostic abnormality is shown in this blood film?

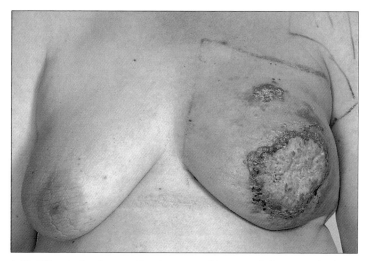

165. What is the abnormality shown on this woman's breast and what treatment is about to be initiated?

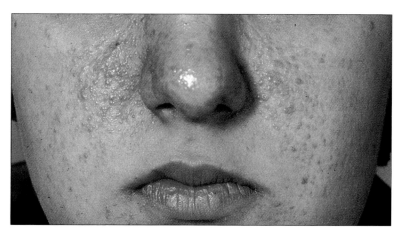

166. This 16-year-old girl presented at the casualty department with an epileptic attack due to failure of drug compliance. What is the cause of her epilepsy and what other features of this disorder would you look for?

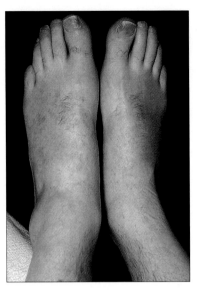

167. This 23-year-old man presented with pain in his left ankle. What abnormality is shown and what is the differential diagnosis? How should the correct diagnosis be established?

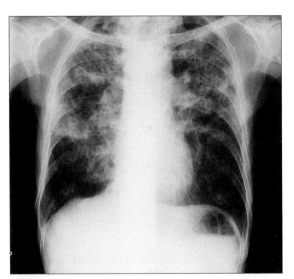

168. This is the x-ray of the chest of a 14-year-old child, who was a recent immigrant from the Far East. The child had weight loss and a persistent cough. What is the diagnosis?

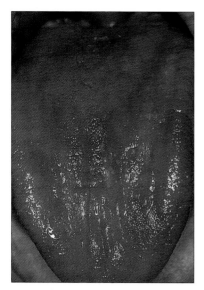

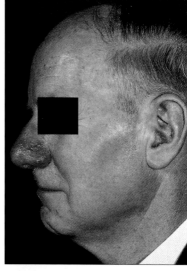

169. What abnormalities are shown in this tongue and what is the likely underlying cause?

170. What abnormality is shown in this picture? What is the differential diagnosis?

171. What does this *x*-ray of the knee of a 26-year-old man show? What was the underlying disease necessitating surgery?

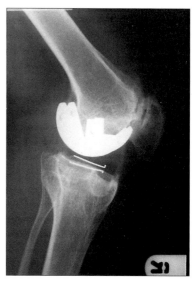

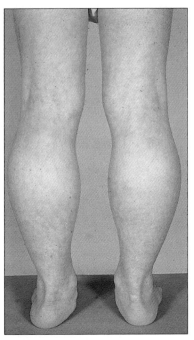

172. This 5-year-old child was brought in for an opinion because of the clumsiness of his gait and difficulties in physical education class. What abnormality is shown? How should the diagnosis be made and what advice is required?

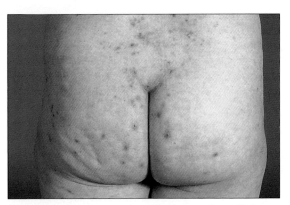

173. This man presented to the dermatology clinic with an intensely itchy rash that particularly involved the elbow, shoulders, buttocks and knees. What is the diagnosis, what further investigations may be indicated and what is the treatment of choice?

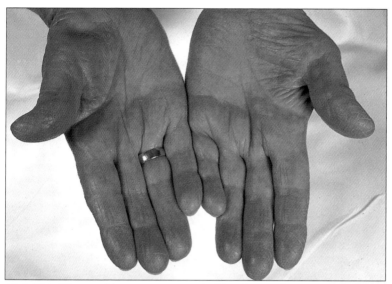

174. This 55-year-old woman presented with pain, numbness and paraesthesia in the fingers of the right hand, which was worst on waking. What abnormality is shown and what is the likely diagnosis? What additional clinical tests should be done and how is the diagnosis confirmed?

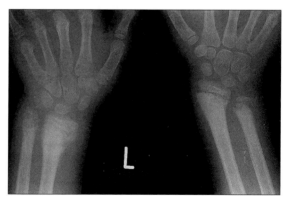

175. This is the *x*-ray of the wrists of a 17-year-old boy. What abnormalities are present and what is the possible diagnosis?

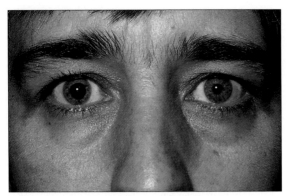

176. This 36-year-old man sought medical advice because his wife had noted that one pupil was smaller than the other. What simple clinical tests should be carried out and what is the disorder?

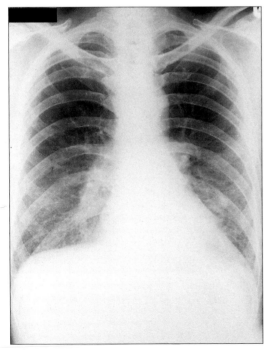

177. This 62-year-old man was sent to the x-ray department with a history of a persistent dry cough. His family doctor had noted that he had marked finger clubbing. What is shown in the x-ray and what additional clinical features will give the clue to the diagnosis?

178. This patient presented for an urgent neurological consultation because of weakness of the right side of the face. What is this syndrome called and what is the mechanism and the prognosis?

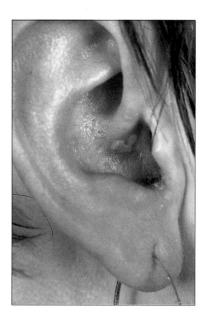

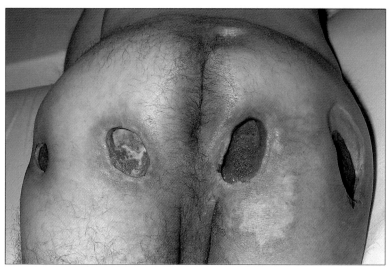

179. What is shown in this picture? What are the complications and what treatment is now required?

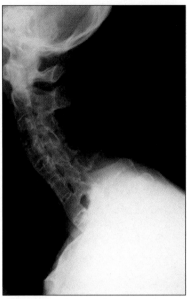

180. What abnormalities are shown in this x-ray and what is the diagnosis?

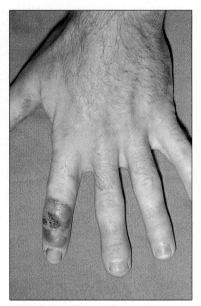

181. What abnormality is shown in the hand of this 28-year-old shepherd? What is it due to?

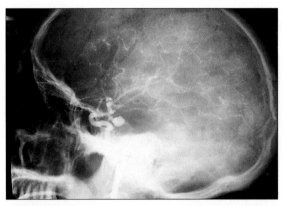

182. This 56-year-old woman presented with sudden-onset severe headache. What kind of x-ray has been done and what does it show?

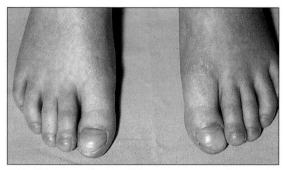

183. What two abnormalities are present in this young patient? What is the likely underlying cause?

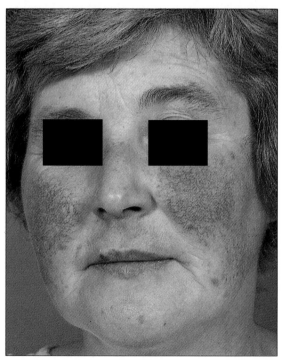

184. This patient has a heart murmur. What is the differential diagnosis?

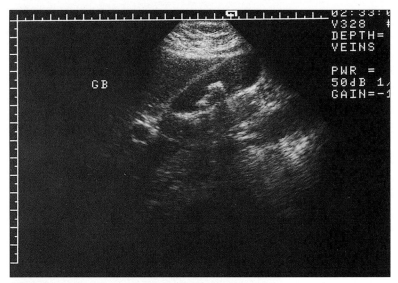

185. What investigation is this and what does it show?

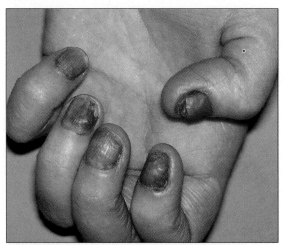

186. This patient has a defect of cell-mediated immunity. What abnormalities are present in her nails and what is the likely cause? What other manifestations may be seen?

187. What abnormalities are seen in this view of a patient's shoulder and upper arm? Name three likely causes.

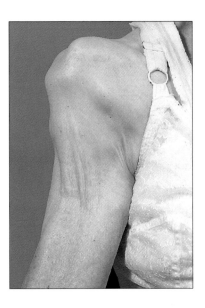

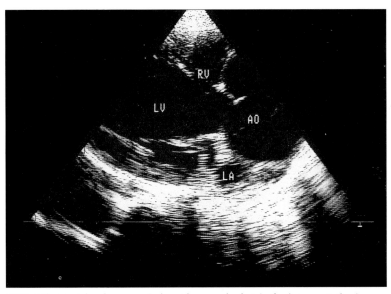

188. What test has been carried out here and what is the interpretation?

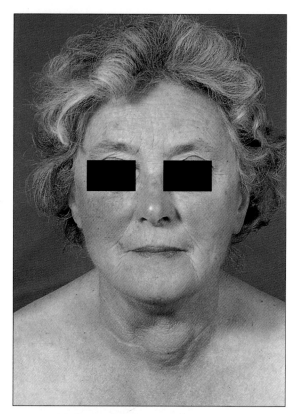

189. What abnormalities are shown in this picture and how should the patient be investigated?

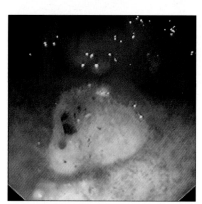

190. What features are shown on this view taken in the stomach? What additional investigations are required and what is the treatment?

191. What two abnormalities are shown in this lateral x-ray of the chest? How may these two abnormalities be linked?

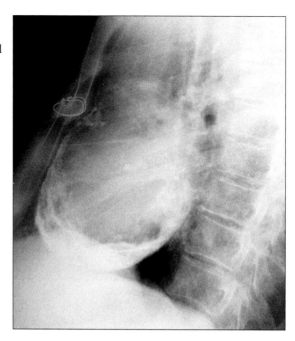

192. What two abnormalities are shown in this picture of the eye of a 56-year-old woman?

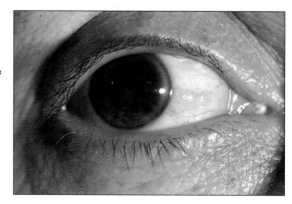

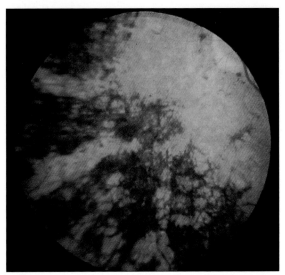

193. This 33-year-old male presented with progressive loss of his peripheral visual fields and night blindness. What changes are present in his visual fields and what is the diagnosis?

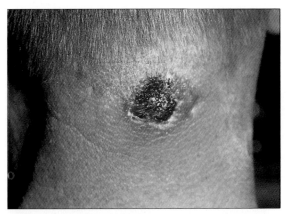

194. This 40-year-old leather worker was admitted with a rapidly growing lesion on his neck. What is the likely diagnosis and how should he be treated?

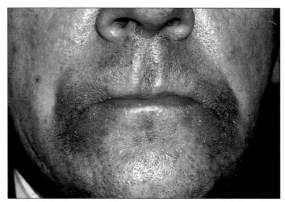

195. This 56-year-old man developed the appearance shown here after using treatment prescribed for seborrhoeic eczema of the face. What is the diagnosis? What is the likely cause? What is the important moral of this story?

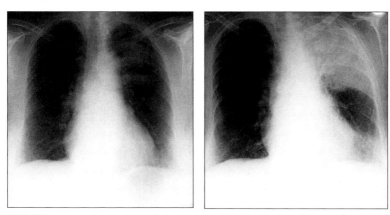

196. These two chest x-rays of the same patient were taken 14 months apart. What do they show, and what is the likely diagnosis?

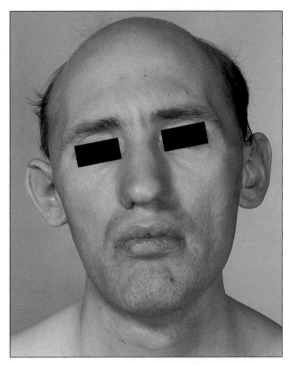

197. This 26-year-old man presented with progressive muscle weakness, clumsiness of his hands and difficulty in walking. What abnormalities are present and what is the likely diagnosis?

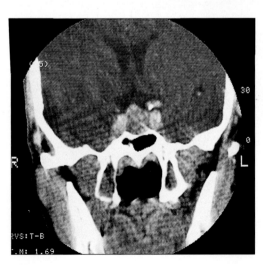

198. What imaging technique has been used to obtain this picture? What abnormality is seen? What complication may result from its local effects?

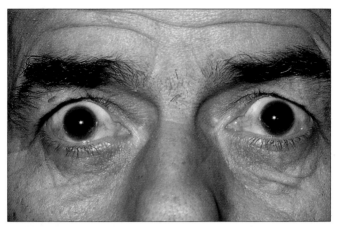

199. During a health screen at work, this 55-year-old man was found to have a biochemical abnormality. He had had a history of peptic ulceration for many years and had been treated with H_2 blockers. There was a history of a renal stone, which he had passed spontaneously. What abnormality is shown here in his eyes, and what disease process does he have? How should this be managed?

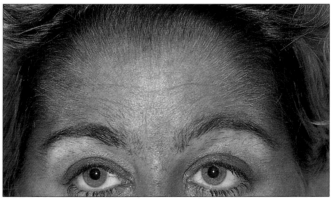

200. This 32-year-old woman was receiving medical treatment for severe renal hypertension. What is the abnormal sign and what is its likely cause?

ANSWERS

1. This man has unilateral exophthalmos (proptosis). As shown here he has lid retraction and he was also demonstrated to have lid lag. Where exophthalmos is unilateral it is essential to exclude the possibility of an orbital or retro-orbital tumour, such as a meningioma on the sheath of the optic nerve, but unilateral or asymmetrical exophthalmos may occur in thyrotoxicosis (Graves' disease). This patient had a small palpable thyroid with no bruit; he was in sinus rhythm but had a resting tachycardia (pulse rate 92/min). The clinical diagnosis was confirmed on finding elevated blood levels of T3 and T4 and undetectable levels of TSH. Control of his thyrotoxicosis with carbimazole reversed the exophthalmos (though the eye signs of Graves' disease do not always respond to antithyroid treatment).

2. This shows extensive psoriasis which has been present at varying degree of severity for the past 20 years in this male patient. The classic features are the erythematous patches with silvery desquamating scales. The classic sites are the extensor surfaces of the knee and the elbow, though the disease may be more widespread. To date, this patient has had no joint symptomatology, although he has the typical nail changes with onycholysis and nail pitting. He has rarely had any obvious lesions on his face or hands; however, he has experienced severe involvement of his scalp. The major effects have been social and emotional. This common disease affects about two per cent of the population, involving males and females equally. There was a positive family history in this case, with his mother being severely affected both in her skin and with psoriatic arthropathy. In this patient there had been episodes of spontaneous remission with acute flare-ups which seem to have been related to alcohol excess. Over the years he has had a variety of treatments some of which occasionally have induced remission. These include dithranol and salicylic acid, corticosteroids in short courses, retinoic acid and PUVA therapy.

3. This man has developed acute gout on a background of previously undiagnosed and untreated chronic gout. The three main abnormalities are:
  (a) Acute swelling of the hand with extreme hyperaemia as shown by the dilated dorsal veins.
  (b) Acute arthritis in the proximal interphalangeal joint of the fourth finger.
  (c) The presence of a deposit of uric acid subcutaneously in the terminal phalanx of the middle finger.
The white, toothpaste-like material was aspirated, and polarized light microscopy showed it to consist of needle-shaped birefringent crystals. The diuretic should be stopped, and a non-steroidal anti-inflammatory drug, such as ibuprofen, should be prescribed. Colchicine is not routinely used now because of its potential side effects. Allopurinol may aggravate the symptoms during the acute attack but it should be used to prevent further attacks once the acute symptoms have settled. Dietary advice should also be given, including a reduction in the intake of meat, especially offal such as liver and kidney. The serum uric acid level should be monitored in the long term and preventive treatment is usually necessary for life.

4. This is a magnetic resonance image in a lady of 38 years from the Shetland Islands, who has a history and clinical features extremely suggestive of multiple sclerosis. The abnormal finding is the "high signal" lesions in the white matter of both hemispheres; these represent areas of demyelination, many of which occur in silent areas of the brain and are not associat-

94

ed with clinical neurological deficits. This woman had sustained an episode of probable optic neuritis many years prior to her current presentation. The current investigation was triggered by an episode of numbness and paraesthesia involving her right leg.

5. This lady shows the typical features of hypothyroidism (myxoedema). It is surprising how often patients are admitted with quite advanced hypothyroidism or with a complication such as myocardial infarction. The problem is that the disease is insidious and the family doctor may not make a diagnosis if he sees the patient regularly, due to the slowly progressive changes. It is worthwhile asking to see a photograph of the patient taken some years earlier; it is then often apparent just how advanced the changes really are. This lady's face is puffy and she has put on weight over the last few years, the hair is coarse and unkempt and she complains of difficulty retaining a perm. The skin is cold and rather coarse and there is some peri-orbital and sub-mandibular puffiness. She has a slight yellow tinge to the skin; this is not due to jaundice but rather to excess circulating beta-carotene. She has become rather hirsute over the years. She had a markedly hoarse voice and her cerebral function was slow. In addition to the obvious facial changes, she had other typical symptoms and signs. Progressive tiredness had prevented her from leaving her house and she had become a virtual recluse. She had put on over 25kg in weight over the last three years and had also become cold intolerant and tended to sit alone at home huddled over an electric fire. As a result she had developed severe erythema ab igne on her legs. She had episodes of confusion, claimed to have lost her appetite and had recently become extremely constipated. Other signs of note were bradycardia (50/min) with some evidence of right heart failure and a small pleural effusion. She complained of tingling of both hands and was found to have bilateral carpal tunnel syndrome. Her peripheral circulation was poor, and she had typical slow-relaxing reflexes. The diagnosis was made by measuring her T4 and her TSH, showing a high level of TSH and a low level of T4. In addition she had a normochronic and normocytic anaemia and a cholesterol level of 8.9mmol/l. Treatment with thyroid hormone must be started at a very low dose in such a patient. She was given thyroxine, 0.025mg per day, and increases were made according to the clinical responses with regular monitoring of her clinical status and ECG for changes suggestive of worsening ischaemia.

6. The picture shows grade four hypertensive retinopathy on the Keith-Wagener scale. There is swelling of the optic nerve head (papilloedema) and the extent of this can be shown by focusing the ophthalmoscope on the optic nerve head and comparing the focus to that of the retinal surface. In addition there are haemorrhages and exudates, arterio-venous nipping and the arteries are extremely constricted. These changes are associated with loss of visual acuity. The older term for this condition is malignant hypertension. The patient's blood pressure was 220/150 mm Hg. It was unknown how long he had been hypertensive as he had not been seen in the practice for several years and had refused offers of routine screening over this time. There was a prior history of an episode of glomerulonephritis at the age of 22 years but this seemed to have settled and he had been discharged from further attendance.

Patients with malignant hypertension should be admitted to hospital for urgent treatment. Bedrest may significantly reduce the blood pressure, but urgent therapy to reduce the blood pressure in a controlled manner is usually necessary. Treatment may include intravenous diazoxide, nitroprusside, hydralazine, atenolol or nifedipine. It is important that the blood pressure is adequately controlled in the long term and that evidence of target organ involvement is looked for. Left ventricular hypertrophy may be revealed by ECG but echocardiography is now the most reliable diagnostic method. Renal function must be evaluated because severe hypertension may lead to renal failure. In addition, possible causes of hypertension should be excluded by appropriate investigations.

7. This is a case of erythema ab igne (Tinker's Tartan). The usual cause is excessive local heat, often from sitting in front of a fire. It is found particularly in the elderly, who sit huddled in front of a coal or electric fire to keep warm. There may also be a degree of ischaemia of the legs and sometimes varicose veins. The end result is thermal damage to capillaries with leakage of red cells to give what looks like a haemorrhagic rash, which eventually becomes brown-stained, as shown here. It may also be seen on the abdomen or chest due to the recurrent application of hot water bottles. The mechanism of capillary damage is similar. It is important to reassure the patient that it is of no significance but it is also wise to exclude other conditions which cause the patient to feel cold, such as hypothyroidism.

8. This patient has the typical features of a right axillary vein thrombosis. The hand, upper arm and shoulder region are swollen and he has pitting oedema from the fingers to the elbow. The arm is also slightly cyanotic and a collateral circulation can be seen round the shoulder and anterior chest wall. On palpation the arm was warm, there was tenderness in the axilla and the inflamed cord of the axillary vein could easily be palpated. There was no tenderness in the neck. The diagnosis was confirmed by upper limb venography. It is important to see if these patients have any external cause of obstruction, in particular, if there is radiological evidence of an accessory rib. It is also important when palpating the neck to see if there is a fibrous band which may obstruct the vein in certain anatomical positions. A search should also be made for any abnormality of coagulation factors, especially proteins C and S and anti-thrombin III; measurement of an anti-cardiolipin antibody should also be carried out. No abnormalities were found and it was presumed that the thrombosis had resulted from postural changes associated with the excessive exercise. It is most unusual for such thrombi to give rise to pulmonary emboli but this has been recorded. The patient should be treated with analgesics, support to the arm and a short course of heparin followed by warfarin for one month. Recurrence of the disease is very unusual.

9. The patient has extensive bilateral apical hilar calcification, resulting from old tuberculosis. An extensive area of shadowing at the right apex can be seen to contain a second, circular shadow. The likely cause of this appearance is an aspergilloma, which has slowly enlarged to its current size within an old tuberculous cavity. *Aspergillus* hyphae were found in the patient's sputum. The treatment of an aspergilloma of this size is surgical.

10. The association of premature grey hair with auto-immune pernicious anaemia is well recognized and this is the most likely clinical diagnosis. Haematological investigation showed this patient to have a macrocytic anaemia with a low white cell count and a low platelet count; the marrow investigation confirmed a megaloblastic picture. The diagnosis of pernicious anaemia was confirmed on finding positive gastric parietal cell auto-antibodies, a low serum B_{12} and normal serum folate, and a high serum iron, iron saturation and ferritin. There is a strong association between pernicious anaemia and carcinoma of the stomach and

this patient had two siblings who had developed carcinoma of the stomach, both of whom had premature grey hair. This man has responded to vitamin B_{12} injections and his haemoglobin level is now normal. Endoscopy showed atrophic gastritis but no evidence of tumour; however, he is on long term surveillance which includes annual endoscopy.

11. There is marked tar staining of the fingers of the right hand. Note that this is often wrongly called nicotine staining, but nicotine is a colourless chemical. The tar stains result from the current smoking of cigarettes and often reflects the fact that the cigarette is smoked right down to the stub. There may also be local burns present. There is also marked finger clubbing. This is always best seen tangentially and in this patient there is marked increased curvature of the nail with loss of the angle between the nail and the nailbed. In addition the tip of the finger is bulbous and the nail "floats" on the nailbed due to the sponginess. The mechanism of development of finger clubbing is not yet known, but it has well-established clinical associations, which include:

Respiratory   Bronchial carcinoma
    Bronchiectasis
    Cystic fibrosis
    Lung abscess
    Emphysema
    Fibrosing alveolitis
    Asbestosis

Cardiological   Cyanotic congenital heart disease
    Infective endocarditis

Gastrointestinal Coeliac disease
    Ulcerative colitis
    Crohn's disease
    Cirrhosis

Idiopathic   Congenital clubbing

12. This is a chylous pleural effusion. The milky appearance is due to the presence of high concentrations of lipids, and the usual cause of this is obstruction of the thoracic duct within the thorax by a primary or secondary carcinoma involving the hilum of the lung.

13. These are the typical lesions of cutaneous larva migrans. The condition is also known as "creeping eruption" or "ground itch". It is the result of contact and penetration of the skin by the larvae of a range of worms, whose normal host is non-human. The larvae cannot develop further in man but migrate in subcutaneous tissue and present with itchy erythematous lesions which may also be vesicular. The range of worms which may cause this reaction include *Ancylostoma brazilinse*, *Ancylostoma canimum*, *Ancylostoma duodenale*, *Necator americanus*, and *Strongyloides stercoralis*. The diagnosis in this case was confirmed by biopsy which showed the larvae of *Strongyloides stercoralis*.

ANSWERS

14. This shows the procedure of pleural biopsy using an Abrams needle. As shown here the needle is inserted into the pleural cavity and may be used to aspirate a pleural effusion. It can then be turned round so that the notch present in the shaft engages with the parietal pleural surface. The inner cutting trocar is then advanced to cut a small biopsy which may include the intercostal muscle as well as pleura and any tumour present. Examples of pleural biopsies are shown in the top right picture. This is an effective way of diagnosing pleural involvement by bronchial carcinoma. The component parts of the Abrams needle are shown in the lower right picture.

15. This is palmar erythema in which there is excessive redness of the skin on both the thenar and hypothenar eminences. The appearances also are present across the top of the palm and in the pulps of the fingers. They suggest the presence of liver disease and may also be called "liver palms", but they can be found in other conditions, including pregnancy, thyrotoxicosis and rheumatoid arthritis and in women who use the oral contraceptive pill. It is thought that in liver disease the changes result from the failure of the liver to degrade oestrogen.

16. The obvious sign is the gross distension of the abdomen due to severe ascites. There are visible superficial dilated veins running up and down her abdomen, originating in the umbilical region. The blood flow in these veins was determined by the two finger test and was from the umbilicus outwards. There is also atrophy of the muscle groups of both upper and lower limbs. This lady had chronic alcoholism which had resulted in multiple admissions to hospital over the years. On this occasion she presented with major haematemesis from known oesophageal varices. It was known from previous admissions that she had had hepatosplenomegaly but the organs could not be felt on this occasion even by ballottement. The patient was icteric, though this is not particularly obvious in this picture, and she had fetor hepaticus. There is a large pressure sore over her left gluteal region associated with her lying stuporose at home. Close examination of her skin showed that she had purpuric spots, and a subsequent platelet count of 35×10^9 per litre confirmed that she had thrombocytopenia. This is probably due to a combination of causes which include hypersplenism, a direct toxic effect of alcohol on the bone marrow and folate deficiency. Note that she is receiving a blood transfusion and that a urinary catheter is in place.

17. These are tendon xanthomata which are deposits of lipids in the extensor tendons of the dorsum of the hand. They are best demonstrated by asking the patient to make a fist. In addition, he had xanthelasmata around both eyes and xanthomas in the Achilles tendons, all of which had been undiagnosed previously. These findings are strongly suggestive of severe hypercholesterolaemia, and a random serum cholesterol level was found to be 9.3mmol/l. It is also important to exclude underlying causes of hypercholesterolaemia, including hypothyroidism, diabetes mellitus and renal disease. Treatment consists of dietary modification, including a reduction of saturated fat intake, a reduction in calorie intake if the patient is overweight, and control of alcohol intake. At this level of cholesterol, drug treatment is also usually needed. This patient was started on simvastatin – an acetyl co-enzyme A reductase inhibitor. The aim is to reduce total serum cholesterol, and to maintain it at a level below 5.2mmol/l. In addition to all these measures, attention has to be paid to the presence of other risk factors for arterial disease, including hypertension, cigarette smoking, diabetes mellitus, stress, body mass index and lack of exercise. Tendon xanthomata are most commonly seen in familial hypercholesterolaemia (Type IIb hyperlipoproteinaemia); the patient's family should be offered appropriate screening with a full profile of total cholesterol, high and low density lipoproteins and triglycerides performed on a fasting sample.

18. This lady has the typical facies of systemic sclerosis. The skin round the mouth is tight and she had been aware of difficulty in opening her mouth, a symptom which had been progressive over some years. The skin is generally waxy and shiny and is particularly puckered around the mouth. She also had some telangiectases round the mouth and on both cheeks. On questioning, she complained of difficulty in swallowing solid foods, but not liquids. Examination of the digits showed telangiectases, the skin was thickened and tethered and cold challenge showed positive Raynaud's phenomenon. There was ulceration of some of the finger pulps and calcinosis was present. There were no alimentary symptoms suggestive of malabsorption and her chest x-ray was normal. She has a common variant of systemic sclerosis known as the CREST syndrome (Calcinosis, Raynaud's phenomenon, Esophageal involvement, Sclerodactyly, Telangiectasia). Investigations showed a slightly raised ESR, and a normochromic, normocytic anaemia. RA latex test and the anti-nuclear antibodies were positive. The anti-scl70 and anti-centromere antibodies were also positive. The treatment of the condition is symptomatic. Because of the severity of the Raynaud's phenomenon, she was treated with a prostacyclin analogue (Iloprost), and she was advised to stop smoking and to wear warm gloves.

19. This patient has a carcinoma of the penis which had caused some local bleeding after sexual intercourse. The patient requires surgical referral for biopsy and a decision about amputation and/or radiotherapy. The man was an active homosexual who was known to be HIV-antibody positive and who continued to have active anal intercourse without using any form of condom protection for either himself or his partners. He was relatively well informed on the risks of venereal infection having read, but ignored, the literature of the Terence Higgins Trust.

The lesion shown does not have the characteristics of typical genital warts which tend to be multiple, fissured, rather pointed lesions which are seen particularly on the frenulum and coronal sulcus as well as the glans. They may also be seen on the shaft of the penis and rarely on the scrotum and in the perineum. They may also occur on the meatus and extend into the urethra.

The lesion shown here is solitary, pearly-white in colour, sessile and firm to the touch. Biopsy confirmed that the lesion was a squamous cell cancer and the patient required local surgery and radiotherapy.

Penile cancer is relatively common and is probably due to the presence of human papilloma virus types 16 and 18. HIV-positive patients have an increased likelihood of a range of cancers and if homosexual these include cancers of anus and penis. Carcinoma of the penis is very unusual in those who have been circumcised early in life.

20. This is an echocardiogram with colour-flow Doppler mapping, in a patient with mild aortic regurgitation. The view is parasternal long axis; the aortic regurgitant jet is coloured blue and is directed posteriorly at an acute angle from the aortic valve, to the right in the picture, back into the left ventricle, to the left in the picture, impinging directly on the anterior mitral valve leaflet, in the centre of the picture, immediately below the blue jet.

ANSWERS

21. This is the typical appearance of senile purpura. The sites affected are usually the extensor surfaces of the forearms and the back of the hands. This is a disease of the elderly in which the skin becomes thin and atrophic and the small venules become superficial and are easily traumatized. The extravasated blood remains purple for many months and gradually fades to leave dark-brown pigmented areas of hemosiderin (age spots). There are no changes in platelets or blood coagulation factors. There is no specific treatment and the patient can be reassured. Similar bruising may be seen in patients of all ages as a result of long-term systemic corticosteroid therapy.

22. There is a swelling in the right axilla which is discrete and about 3cm in diameter. It is not attached to skin or to deeper tissue, is non-tender and has all the characteristics of a lymph node. Similar nodes were found in the other axilla, and bilaterally in the neck and inguinal regions. In this patient both epitrochlear lymph nodes were also felt. In addition, this lady had skin purpura, ulceration of the tonsils, and massive splenomegaly. Examination of her peripheral blood film suggested that she had chronic myeloid leukaemia and this diagnosis was confirmed on bone marrow aspiration.

23. This is a computed tomogram (CT) of the thorax at the level of the great vessels. The major abnormality is shown posteriorly on the left side. This is a large empyema that formed in a patient admitted in the first instance with pneumonia. Aspirated pus grew *Staphylococcus aureus*, which was resistant to penicillin. Combination antibiotic therapy resulted in rapid improvement.

24. This young man has acute tonsillitis, with massive enlargement of both tonsils, which are coated with a membrane that is not easily removed. He has an accumulation of saliva in his mouth due to the pain of swallowing. In addition there are purpuric spots on the palate and some local ulcers. These appearances are typical of infectious mononucleosis (IM), although other diagnoses must be considered, including streptococcal tonsillitis and HIV infection. This patient had lymph node enlargement in the cervical, axillary and inguinal regions and splenomegaly. The diagnosis of IM was confirmed on the finding of abnormal lymphocytes in his peripheral blood smear and a positive Monospot test. His liver function tests were normal and HIV antibody test was negative.

25. The dominant features of the fundus are multiple dot and blot haemorrhages and hard exudates in all areas of the retina. The visible arteries and veins are normal and there is no evidence of increased light reflex or AV nipping. This is a typical appearance of diabetic retinopathy. There is no evidence of retinal vessel proliferation.

26. This girl has a partial oculomotor (IIIrd) nerve palsy and as can be seen, she has ptosis on the right. The right eye also looks downwards and to the right. The pupil showed no reaction to light or accommodation. The oculomotor nerve has a long course within the cranium, passes close to the posterior communicating artery and then along the lateral wall of the cavernous sinus. It is therefore at risk of damage due to an expanding aneurysm of one of its related arteries. Such a lesion is best diagnosed by cerebral angiography as it is a difficult area to visualize on CT or MRI scanning.

27. These lesions are typical of erythema nodosum, in which tender, painful, purplish-red nodules appear, usually on the shins, thighs and occasionally on the upper arms. They fade slowly over several weeks leaving a bruised area, and they do not ulcerate. The commonest cause in the United Kingdom is now reaction to drugs, and sulphonamides are the most commonly identified precipitants of the disease. In many patients no cause may be identified. In addition, these lesions may appear in association with many other diseases (see below). There may be accompanying malaise, fatigue, fever and joint pains. No specific treatment is required; treatment should be orientated towards the primary disease. Usually the lesions disappear within a few days but occasionally they are persistent over several months. Common causes of erythema nodosum are:

Infections: Bacterial – streptococcus, tuberculosis, brucellosis, leprosy, yersinia
Mycoplasma
Rickettsia
Chlamydia
Viral
Fungal – histoplasmosis, coccidioidomycosis
Drugs: Sulphonamides, oral contraceptives, penicillin
Systemic Diseases: Sarcoidosis, inflammatory bowel disease, Beçhet's disease.
Pregnancy

28. The patient has bilateral double (duplex) ureters, with associated duplication of the renal pelves. The normal ureters can be seen to enter the bladder in the normal position, while the ectopic ureters, draining the ectopic, upper poles of the kidneys, enter the bladder below and medial to the normal ureters (in this view, this is only clearly seen on the patient's left). Double ureters may be a harmless anomaly, but they are sometimes associated with abnormal urinary tract function and recurrent ascending urinary tract infections, which may lead on to chronic renal failure if untreated. Occasionally the ecopic ureter may open into the urethra (or the ejaculatory duct in a male), with further risks of dysfunction and infection.

29. This *x*-ray shows multiple cannonball shadowing, typical of multiple secondary deposits in both lungfields. There is also a small effusion at the left costophrenic angle. The heart shadow is enlarged and the appearances suggest that there are secondaries in the pericardium and that part of the enlargement of the cardiac shadow is due to pericardial effusion. This appearance is seen with secondaries from a primary in various organs; prime suspects include the kidneys, testes, thyroid and, in females, breasts and ovaries.

30. This is a fine needle aspiration of a thyroid swelling in a woman who has previously undergone thyroidectomy. Initial investigation of such patients should be biochemical, to determine whether the patient is hyperthyroid. Radioisotope scans demonstrate whether the nodule is "hot", i.e. producing thyroid hormone, or "cold", in which case a cyst or tumour is a possibility. The anatomical structure can be investigated by ultrasound and the cytology of the lesion is determined by aspiration. This is a straightforward technique under local anaesthesia and is highly successful in obtaining cells for cytological examination. It is the investigation of choice in suspected thyroid carcinoma.

ANSWERS

31. This is acute skin necrosis, which is usually of sudden onset and may be haemorrhagic in nature and rapidly followed by extensive sloughing of the skin. The usual sites are over the breast and abdomen. The cause is protein C deficiency which may be congenital or acquired. Protein C is a liver-produced coagulation protein which is necessary for the normal integrity of blood vessels. Administration of warfarin to patients inhibits the production by the liver of coagulation factors II, VII, IX, and X and also of protein C. Protein C deficiency results in microthrombosis and necrosis of skin as shown in this picture. Warfarin should be withdrawn, and anticoagulation continued with heparin. Skin grafting may be required in the affected area.

32. This picture shows a swollen oedematous left leg which was warm to the touch and tender in the calf; the tenderness extended right up into the thigh on the medial side. The thickened inflamed femoral vein was easily palpable. These clinical features in the context of a patient who has had major surgery, especially in association with carcinoma, suggests an iliofemoral deep-vein thrombosis. As there are many conditions that mimic this situation it is imperative that the diagnosis be confirmed by a "gold-standard" test such as venography or ultrasound. Here ultrasound showed thrombus occluding the femoral vein. Treatment is with conventional anti-coagulants; the patient was initially heparinized to give an activated partial thromboplastin time (APTT) of twice the normal and at the same time warfarin was commenced in a loading dose of 10mg followed by 5mg/day. After two or three days of heparin the warfarin should have achieved a maximal effect and warfarin dosage is adjusted over the next three months to maintain the international normalized ratio (INR) between 2.5 and 3.5. Other initial treatment should include the use of an analgesic to relieve discomfort and the use of support hose. Note the plaque of psoriasis on the patient's right leg, which was a coincidental finding.

33. In most intravenous drug abusers, lack of hygiene associated with venous access results in local thrombophlebitis. This girl had run out of easily accessible arm veins and had taken to injecting into her femoral vein. There was a lack of any sterile procedures and she had developed an abscess in her groin as a result of this. Subsequent culture grew *Staphylococcus aureus*. In addition she had been injecting a range of drugs including crushed-up tablets of temazepam. The appearance of her foot suggests multiple small emboli which may be due to the insoluble excipient in the tablet or to septic emboli from the groin abscess. A similar appearance could result from infective endocarditis – a common complication in intravenous drug abusers.

34. This picture shows the typical appearances of diffuse gum hypertrophy, most commonly associated with the long-term use of phenytoin for the control of epileptic seizures. The mechanism of this hypertrophy is not known, but it is often associated with a degree of dental caries and plaque formation as shown here. The patient requires dental hygiene care and a decision was made to convert him to an anticonvulsant which does not lead to this complication (sodium valproate).

35. This *x*-ray shows the typical appearances of pulmonary abscess in the right mid-zone, with at least two fluid filled cavities. The initial pathology almost certainly was associated with an aspiration pneumonia due to his comatose state. The patient was ill with a high

swinging fever and was treated initially with intravenous antibiotics and had a stormy conva-
lescence complicated by the appearance of a deep vein thrombosis.

36. This man had disseminated intravascular coagulation due to septicaemia with
Staphylococcus aureus. The diagnosis of DIC was made on the basis of low platelet count
(30×10^9/l), the presence of high amounts of fibrinogen degradation products (FDPs), and
prolonged prothrombin and partial thromboplastin times. In addition Factor VIII and
Factor V were low. The purpura is not only due to the thrombocytopenia but also to the
presence of the FDPs which interfere with platelet function as well as the polymerization of
fibrin. Supportive treatment should be combined with the intravenous administration of
appropriate antibiotics.

37. The tibia is anteriorly bowed and thickened. The normal bone architecture is totally lost
and has been replaced with areas of lucency and areas of increased bone density. There is
also destruction of the knee joint due to the loss of the normal articular anatomy. No frac-
tures are seen within the bone and there is no evidence of sarcomatous change. This is the
typical finding of Paget's disease of bone (osteitis deformans). It is to be noticed as an incidental finding that there is also arterial calcification present. This patient's dominant clinical
problem was bone pain of a constant nature unrelieved by rest or by changing posture.
Paget's disease is a common problem in the elderly and it often requires no treatment.
However, because of the pain this man was treated with diphosphonate.

38. The patient has skin tags and proctoscopy showed small non-bleeding haemorrhoids. The
prominent finding is, however, a large ulcer at the anal margin with an infected base. The
rolled edge was firm and pearly coloured. Biopsy of the lesion showed that this was an anal carcinoma and treatment was radical surgery, due to its advanced nature.

39. This is the foot of a 62-year-old patient who was known to have had mature onset diabetes (non-insulin dependent, Type II) and who had initially been controlled on diet alone
for five years. In the last three years he had required an oral agent (gliclazide). He had
neglected his care and had often defaulted from clinic attendance. On this occasion he was
seen with an obvious ulcer on his great toe which was painless but infected. It was punched
out and the underlying tissues were clearly exposed. There was diabetic neuropathy present
and there was severe disease of the small vessels to the feet. X-ray of the toe showed no bone
involvement. The ulcer eventually healed with expert chiropody, control of the infection and
tight diabetic control.

40. This is a thyroid scan that has been carried out using ^{99m}Tc. The vascularity of the thyroid leads to a clear image by this technique. Here, the right lobe of the thyroid is enlarged
compared to the left and there is a very large "cold" area, in which the blood supply is
reduced. Such a cold nodule requires further investigation, initially by an aspiration needle
biopsy. About 20 per cent of such lesions are carcinomatous, and the diagnosis can usually
be made by cytological investigation of the aspirate.

41. This marrow is megaloblastic but in this picture it is not particularly cellular. This
patient had a haemoglobin of 6g/dl with a white cell count of 1×10^9/l and a platelet count

ANSWERS

of $60 \times 10^9/l$. The megaloblasts are larger than the typical erythroblast and have a fine, open stippled chromatin pattern. There is a dissociation between nuclear and cytoplasmic maturation so that the resultant red cells are larger than normal (they have a high MCV) and they are found in the peripheral blood as macrocytes. This patient had pernicious anaemia. This is an autoimmune disorder that results from the immune destruction of the parietal cells of the gastric mucosa, which leads to a deficiency in the production of intrinsic factor necessary for the absorption of B^{12}. Pernicious anaemia is commonly associated with prematurely grey hair and with a personal or family history of other single-organ autoimmune disorders, such as those of the thyroid and adrenal. The patient had a low serum B^{12} assay with a positive two-stage Schilling test and a normal folate. In addition, the serum iron and percentage saturation were high and there was a high level of indirect bilirubin, which is a reflection of the ongoing haemolysis of cells before they leave the marrow. The serum total LDH was also elevated due to haemolysis. Such patients rapidly respond to B^{12} and it is important to remember to give iron therapy simultaneously as they may otherwise rapidly become iron depleted.

42. This is toxic epidermal necrolysis (Lyell's disease). It is also known as the scalded skin syndrome and is most commonly a reaction to staphylococcal infection. Staphylococcal toxin produces epidermal cleavage in the Malpighian layer of the skin. There is often a prodrome of short duration before the skin starts to be shed. It is usual to treat the patient with steroids and anti-staphylococcal antibiotics, but there is little evidence that these significantly change the course of the disease when it has developed to this stage. However, antibiotic treatment may help to prevent the spread of bacteria to other children. A similar reaction may occur following immunization and as a complication of treatment with drugs such as sulphonamides.

43. This is gingivostomatitis, due to infection with *Herpes simplex* virus type I. This 15-year-old boy presented with lower-grade fever and developed lesions on his lips and buccal mucosa. They were extremely painful and were associated with increased salivation and with coating of the tongue. Initially, multiple vesicles formed, then coalesced and ruptured to leave painful necrotic ulcers. He had a general systemic upset with elevation of the white cell count. This infection is often self-limiting and these lesions disappeared in two weeks. It is important to encourage a high fluid intake because of the fever, but pain in the mouth may make this difficult. Administration of acyclovir shortens the course of the disease.

44. This lady had been diagnosed as having Graves' disease and had bilateral exophthalmos. Despite adequate treatment of her thyrotoxicosis, the eye signs became more marked with evidence of infiltrative ophthalmopathy. In this situation the exophthalmos is still present (as can be confirmed by the use of an exophthalmometer), and there is lid and conjunctival oedema. The extraocular muscles are infiltrated and there is limitation of the ocular movements. She had difficulty closing the lids over the cornea especially in the right eye and this had resulted in conjunctival and corneal irritation. In addition she had diplopia and as can be seen there is a divergence of the left eye. Orbital ultrasound and orbital computed tomography showed extreme infiltration of the extraocular muscles. Exposure keratopathy should be treated with ocular lubricants, and surgical tarsorrhaphy may be necessary as a temporary measure. The progressive exophthalmos and optic nerve damage may respond to systemic steroids, but surgical decompression of the optic nerve sheath may be required.

45. This man has major wasting of the small muscles of the hand, particularly of the first dorsal interosseous of his left hand. Above the wrist is a scar – the result of a deep cut from broken glass that damaged the ulnar nerve. Characteristically muscle weakness and atrophy predominate in this situation and the major disability is in the performance of fine movements involving the thumb and fingers. This patient also had some numbness of the little finger and along the ulnar border of the palm.

46. As the patient is generally unwell and the lesion has grown quickly the possibility of a reticulosis or a secondary carcinomatous deposit should be considered. On examination the patient seemed pale, was probably anaemic and looked unwell. He had a low-grade fever but the dominant features were the presence of diffuse lymphadenopathy with small painless rubbery lymph nodes in the cervical, axillary and inguinal regions. In addition the spleen tip could be felt 2cm below the costal margin. The skin lesion on his back was brownish/purple in colour, seemed warm to the touch, was elevated above the skin surface and was non-tender. Biopsy of the lesion is the quickest method of making a definitive diagnosis. Biopsy of lymph nodes and of the back lesion showed the typical appearance of a non-Hodgkin's lymphoma of the histiocytic type; that is, the malignant cells are large and irregular with abundant cytoplasm; some of the cells are multinucleated and resemble the Reed-Sternberg cell. X-ray of his chest showed mediastinal lymphadenopathy bilaterally. CT scan confirmed the presence of splenomegaly and showed multiple lymph node enlargement within the abdomen. The liver was normal. Advanced disease (stage IVB) requires aggressive chemotherapy with a combination of drugs, which may include cyclophosphamide, vincristine, prednisolone and procarbazine. Allopurinol should be given to inhibit the elevation of uric acid that may result from tissue catabolism.

47. This picture shows acute, severe conjunctivitis. The additional clinical information which was obtained was that the oedema which developed on the palms and soles was followed by desquamation of the skin of the fingers and toes. The patient also had proteinuria, a normochromic anaemia and leucocytosis. No viral or bacterial infection was found on extensive investigation. The clinical picture is that of Kawasaki's disease (mucocutaneous lymph node syndrome), a disease of unknown aetiology which is usually of acute onset and then is self-limiting after a benign course. It occurs in epidemics worldwide and is probably often missed or misdiagnosed. In about half the patients there is electrocardiographic evidence of pericarditis or myocarditis and there is a mortality of about 1% in the later stages of the illness due to coronary artery involvement by localized arteritis with bead-like aneurysms forming. Death from myocardial infarction or heart failure associated with ischaemia may result. Most patients require no specific treatment except for symptomatic management. However, if there is evidence of myocarditis they should receive aspirin, a broad-spectrum antibiotic and anticoagulants. There is no evidence that steroids have any place in the management and studies have shown that patients treated with steroids do significantly less well than those who are not.

ANSWERS

48. This is a double-contrast barium enema and shows multiple diverticula involving the whole colon but particularly the sigmoid colon (diverticulosis). There is some narrowing of the lumen with evidence of sinus formation between adjacent areas of diverticulitis. This has almost certainly resulted from local abscess formation. It is important to exclude the presence of an associated colonic neoplasm, so colonoscopy, and biopsy, should be undertaken. Long-term management is conservative with appropriate dietary alteration, usually including an increase in the amount of fibre in the diet. Iron therapy may be needed to correct the iron-deficient anaemia and occasionally surgery may be required.

49. These two pictures show marked oesophagitis and in the picture on the right (b) there is also a large ulcer. This has resulted from the reflux of gastric juice containing hydrochloric acid and pepsin, causing erosion and inflammation of the mucosal squamous epithelium. The basic cause is probably a defect in oesophageal motility, which is often associated with a hiatus hernia. In this woman there was a rolling hiatus hernia, probably related to her gross obesity and smoking habit.

The dominant symptoms were burning retrosternal pain, which was exacerbated on lying down, especially in bed, and on stooping to work in the garden, and also reflux of bitter acid after meals.

Symptomatic relief was obtained by following advice on posture, weight control and stopping smoking, and medication with antacids containing alginates and a local anaesthetic. In addition an H_2 blocker or a proton-pump blocker may be valuable, especially at night, to prevent nocturnal acid reflux.

Biopsy of the ulcer was undertaken to ensure that it was not malignant.

50. This woman has long-standing varicose ulceration, affecting the medial borders of both legs. As a young woman she had bilateral venous thromboses following pregnancy. Over the years she had multiple episodes of discomfort in the veins of both legs and had developed varicose veins, which had been operated on several times. The end result is known as postphlebitic syndrome. As can be seen, there is an area of a woody, hard induration that is brown coloured due to leakage of red cells and the subsequent accumulation of hemosiderin. The centre of this area has ulcerated on numerous occasions and healing is only achieved with great difficulty. The acute treatment consists of the use of graduated support hose, elevation of the limb to reduce the hydrostatic pressure, appropriate antiseptic treatment to remove the infection within the ulcer and allow it to heal, and occasionally the use of full thickness skin grafting. However, these ulcers are liable to recur and may be a severe problem for the patient.

51. This is herpes zoster (shingles) which is due to infection with the *Varicella zoster* virus. This virus may lie dormant in the dorsal root ganglia for many years before being activated by some intercurrent illness. Here the maxillary branch of the 5th nerve has been involved and the rash is well demarcated, extending from the mid-line to the ear and into the mouth. At this stage in the progression of the rash, the vesicles have all ruptured and have left scaly, scabby lesions on the cheek. Pain has been one of the dominant features and has prevented the patient from shaving. He has some conjunctivitis and his left pupil is dilated. Acyclovir given orally may be of value in reduction of the duration and severity of the disease and may also prevent the longer-term complication of post-herpetic neuralgia. Appropriate analgesics are required for pain control.

52. The clinical history elicited in this patient is of long standing chronic bronchitis with emphysema (chronic obstructive pulmonary diseas: COPD). He had been a life-long heavy smoker and also worked in a local shipyard as a general labourer. His main problem had been winter bronchitis in which he produced thick tenacious sputum virtually all the time which was frequently infected. The PA view of the chest shows hyperinflation of both lungs with depression of both cusps of the diaphragm and the characteristic long thin mediastinum of emphysema. The right diaphragm is tented, which is a reflection of previous basal chest infections, and there is a left pleural effusion. There are old calcified lesions at the hila and both apices, probably reflecting previous healed tuberculosis. The right lateral of the chest shows hyperinflation and alteration of the normal architecture of the chest wall (barrel chest).

53. This pateint has pompholyx, a variant of eczema involving recurrent episodes of vesiculation on the palms, sides of the fingers and/or soles of the feet. The condition is usually characterised by periods of remission and relapse. Relapse may be the result of exposure to heat or of emotional stress. Pompholyx of the hands may sometimes be a remtoe response (and 'id reaction') to fungal infection of the feet. More controversially, it has beeen suggested that pompholyx may sometimes result from the ingestion of small quantities of nickel (possibly disolved from cooking utensils) by nickel-sensitised patients. Treatment usually involves the use of emollients and topical steroids. In severe cases, occlusive or even systemic steroid treatment may be necessary, and secondary infection may also require antimicrobial treatment.

54. This is the Stevens-Johnson syndrome. As can be seen, the rash is similar to that of erythema multiforme. Many of the skin lesions start with vesiculation and the formation of larger bullae which rupture to give this appearance. In addition, she has oral and genital ulceration and severe conjunctivitis. This condition can be the end result of a variety of triggers ranging from infections with *Mycoplasma pneumoniae*, *Herpes simplex* virus and a range of other viruses to drug therapy, especially with sulphonamides. In many patients, however, no cause is found. In most of the patients the disease is self limiting, but in severe cases systemic steroids may be helpful (though this has been challenged recently) and local applications of steroid eyedrops may be required for conjunctivitis. If any treatable cause of infection is considered to be the trigger, then specific antibiotic therapy should be directed towards this. Intravenous fluids and nasogastric feeding may be required if there is severe ulceration of the nasopharynx.

55. This straight *x*-ray of the abdomen shows multiple-faceted gallstones filling the gallbladder. In addition, stones have migrated into the cystic duct and are impacted in the common bile duct. The patient had obstructive jaundice with the typical biochemical and clinical picture. In addition there is evidence of air in the ducts, almost certainly as a result of bacterial infection. Such patients are often extremely ill with the metabolic defect being compounded by septicaemia and endotoxic shock. The patient required resuscitation, circulatory support and therapy with antibiotics active against Gram-negative organisms. When the general condition improves, the gall bladder and any stones that have migrated should be removed. This may often be done by limited access surgery in association with ERCP.

56. This shows the typical appearances of Henoch-Schönlein purpura – a hypersensitivity reaction that presents as a diffuse vasculitis. There may be a previous history of upper respiratory infection, especially in children. It is probable that the purpura is an immune response to some unknown antigen. Purpura is especially seen on the upper thighs and buttocks; the purpuric spots are often raised and palpable and may appear in crops. As shown in this slide, trauma to the skin, for example by the wearing of a tight belt, may induce the purpuric lesions. Acute intestinal bleeding and nephritis often accompany the obvious skin lesions. In most cases the disease remits spontaneously in about a week, but there may be a recurrence after some months, especially after upper respiratory infections. Renal involvement presents with microscopic haematuria and disturbance of renal function. The serum IgA levels are often elevated and renal biopsy shows mesangial proliferative glomerulonephritis. Electron microscopy confirms the presence of mesangial deposits of IgA. There is no specific treatment.

57. This man had a *Mycoplasma pneumoniae* infection which he had acquired during one of the four-year cycles of this disease. The dominant symptom of his illness was persistent coughing. The x-ray showed an area of consolidation in the left mid-zone near the hilum. Despite his infection he had a white cell count of only 12×10^9/l but his ESR was 80mm in the first hour. Skin manifestations of this organism are relatively uncommon but include vesicular eruptions (as shown), erythema multiforme and erythema nodosum. There is also a reported association with Stevens-Johnson syndrome. In addition to the skin, the nervous system, heart and joints may also be involved, although they were not in this particular patient. Treatment is usually with erythromycin or a tetracycline.

58. This lady has developed cavernous sinus thrombosis. As can be seen, there is an inflammatory reaction involving the left eye, which is swollen, with a swollen lid, and almost closed. Inflammation extends upwards over the forehead and over the left cheek and there is also chemosis. The swelling shown here suggests that the ophthalmic vein has been obstructed as it enters the cavernous sinus. The eyeball was painful and there was photophobia so that examination of the fundus was limited, but it was thought that she also had papilloedema. Movement of the eyeball was also limited by pain. Paralysis of the extraocular muscles is a well-recognized complication. The pupil was dilated due to involvement of the parasympathetic innervation. The prime cause was not found but was presumed to be an adjacent focus of infection. The usual sites of infection are the middle ear, the maxillary sinus, the nose and the periorbital region of the face. Infection may also spread from related thrombophlebitis in other venous sinuses. The most common infecting organism is *Staphylococcus aureus*. Treatment is directed at control of the infection and should include an antibiotic directed against the *Staphylococcus*. In addition anticonvulsants may be used, as epileptiform seizures are common. There is no evidence that anticoagulation is of value and it may carry a risk of inducing haemorrhage. Cavernous sinus thrombosis carries a significant mortality, but recovery is usually complete in patients who survive.

59. This is pyoderma gangrenosum, a well-recognised complication of ulcerative colitis. The lesions usually arise as inflammatory pustules, as shown in the lower of the two lesions. The upper lesion rapidly progressed and broke down to form a large sloughing necrotic ulcer, the edge of which is undermined and has this typical purplish appearance. Despite the obvious inflammation the lesion was not particularly painful. It persisted for several weeks despite the use of local steroids and minocycline. It then responded rapidly to systemic corticosteroids. The dominant histological feature is an intense cellular infiltrate mainly of polymorphs. No organism has been implicated in its aetiology, although it is usual to find skin contaminants. Pyoderma gangrenosum may also be found in a variety of other conditions including rheumatoid arthritis and related arthropathies, acute leukaemia and hyperviscosity syndromes such as multiple myeloma and Waldenström's macroglobulinaemia.

60. This man has gynaecomastia. It is probably due to cyproterone acetate, an anti-androgen which is used in the treatment of prostatic carcinoma. It is important to remember that the diagnosis of gynaecomastia in a man depends on the presence of palpable enlarged breast tissue. It must not be confused with the pseudo-gynaecomastia which is often found in the obese male. A wide range of possible causes of gynaecomastia include liver disease, hyperthyroidism, oestrogen-producing tumours, carcinoma of the male breast and starvation followed by refeeding. Drugs that have been involved include oestrogens and other drugs with an oestrogenic effect such as digoxin, verapamil, cannabis and diamorphine; anti-androgens such as spironolactone and cyproterone; gonadotrophins; cimetidine; and a range of cytotoxics. It is important to explain to patients who require therapy known to induce gynaecomastia what the side effects may be, and to ensure they understand them. Gynaecomastia may also occur physiologically in the male at neonatal, pubertal and geriatric stages of life.

61. This is a case of cervicofacial actinomycosis due to infection with *Actinomyces israelii* which is an anaerobic filamentous bacterium. It may be found as a commensal in the mouth and in the intestine, and probably gained access via the abscess or the dental socket. The patient was aware of a progressive swelling below the jaw which was only slightly painful. She had low-grade fever at this time and general malaise. The lesion ruptured to discharge yellowish pus, leaving this indolent ulcer that continued to discharge yellow "sulphur granule" pus. There was no relevant associated lymphadenopathy. Treatment is with a prolonged course of high-dose intravenous penicillin, amoxycillin, erythromycin or a cephalosporin.

62. This is a two-dimensional echocardiogram in the long-axis view from the apex through the left ventricle and both atria. It shows prolapse of the posterior cusp of the mitral valve into the left atrium anteriorly. Mitral valve prolapse is common but in some patients it is associated with progressive heart disease, usually presenting as heart failure. It is often also associated with arrhythmias and there is a significant incidence of sudden death. In younger people congenital causes should be looked for, in particular Marfan's syndrome. Mitral valve prolapse may also be found in patients with ischaemic heart disease and rheumatic heart disease.
It is important to remember that such patients are at risk of endocarditis after dental extraction or other invasive procedures and appropriate prophylaxis should be offered to them at such times.

ANSWERS

63. The obvious abnormalities in the picture include the degree of skin pigmentation, which is partly melanin and partly icterus. The patient is also clearly jaundiced on inspection of the sclerae. She has marked xanthelasmata in both lower lids and has marked bilateral arcus cornealis. There is a patch of vitiligo across the bridge of the nose. This patient had been attending the clinic for many years with primary biliary cirrhosis (PBC), which is usually associated with hyperlipidaemia, and thus with xanthelasmata and arcus cornealis. Jaundice and melanin deposition are also consequences of PBC. Vitiligo is not the result of PBC, but is often associated with it and with other organ-specific autoimmune disorders.

64. The obvious lesion is a large goitre. Causes include dietary iodine deficiency, dyshormogenetic goitre, physiological demand in pregnancy, thyroiditis, and neoplasia. The patient also has some of the features of hypothyroidism, with oedema of the skin of the face, especially around the eyes. There is no loss of hair on the head or on the eyebrows, but she had a marked bradycardia, a hoarse voice and cold dry skin. There was a family history of goitre and this was considered to be a dyshormonogenetic goitre. She was treated with thyroxine, but surgery may be required for the goitre, especially if retrosternal extension and/or tracheal compression occur.

65. The chest *x*-ray shows the heart shadow to be generally enlarged and globular. The most likely cause is a pericardial effusion. This may be confirmed by echocardiography and the effusion aspirated for diagnostic or therapeutic purposes.

66. This is rubella (German measles) which is normally a self-limiting, rather trivial illness and is now not commonly seen in this age group due to the general availability of vaccination. However, a significant percentage of the female population have not been vaccinated. The importance of the disease is that it may affect the fetus in early pregnancy so it is important to ensure that the patient is not pregnant. Other members of the family should be warned about the risk of fetal abnormalities, and if any are pregnant, prophylaxis with hyperimmune globulin should be offered. If the index case is pregnant, the accuracy of the clinical diagnosis must be confirmed by culturing the virus from throat swabs or urine and also by measuring the increasing serum antibody titre. In a pregnant patient with confirmed rubella, termination of pregnancy should be offered, as the risk of severe congenital abnormality, especially cardiac disease and deafness, is very high.

67. This is circinate balanitis, which is characteristic of Reiter's disease. The lesions on the penis started as small discrete oval red maculae that became confluent. In addition, the patient had vesicular lesions in the buccal mucosa. Treatment was with non-steroidal anti-inflammatories; the eye, genital and mouth lesions settled rapidly while joint swelling and discomfort was still present some months later. From his past history it was apparent that the patient had had a urogenital infection; although no culture was taken at the time it is likely to have been caused by *Chlamydia trachomatis*, which has been shown to be the progenitor of Reiter's disease of genital origin. Reiter's disease may also follow gastrointestinal infections, when other organisms, including *Shigella*, *Salmonella* and *Yersinia* may be cultured from stools. Tissue type HLA-B27 predisposes men to Reiter's disease following these infections.

68. This barium swallow shows that the patient has extensive oesophageal varices. This man had been a chronic alcoholic, but this was his first medical presentation. He had clinical evidence of portal hypertension with splenomegaly and superficial veins on his abdominal wall. He was also slightly icteric with a tender liver felt 3cm below the right costal margin. The veins in the oesophagus and stomach were injected with a sclerosant via the endoscope once the acute episode had settled and his coagulation abnormality had been corrected.

69. This girl has contact dermatitis, and the most likely cause is allergy to nickel. The problem started with the piercing of her ears and the implanting of the ear-ring as shown. Contact dermatitis to nickel is an allergy that affects about 10 per cent of European women and may appear at the site of jewellery contact, particularly bracelets, necklaces and ear-rings, and also at the point of fastening of undergarments such as brassieres and corsets. Some patients may have problems even from contact with nickel in saucepans or door-handles. A patch test can be used to confirm the diagnosis, and avoidance of nickel contact is the only preventive treatment.

70. There is shortening of the middle finger of the left hand, due to an abnormality in the third metacarpal, which is approximately a centimetre shorter than the others. This is a feature of pseudo-hypoparathyroidism, which is caused by a defect at the parathyroid hormonal (PTH) receptor level. Such patients often have a characteristic biochemical profile with a low-serum calcium, raised inorganic phosphate, a usually normal alkaline phosphatase and a raised PTH. There are commonly other skeletal abnormalities including short stature, short neck, abnormal dentition and shortening of metatarsals and metacarpals. There may also be a degree of mental retardation.

71. This patient has developed ischaemic necrosis of the skin of the dorsum of the foot following an attempt at injection of contrast medium for venography. Some hypertonic contrast media are extremely irritant and this is the end result of injection into the soft tissues. Such lesions may require plastic surgery.

72. This is a gross example of barber's rash due to *Streptococcus pyogenes* invasion of the hair follicles, producing typical vesicular and crusted lesions. Blood culture was negative but the patient responded to systemic treatment with penicillin.

73. The appearance of this patient's lips, tongue and skin suggests hereditary haemorrhagic telangiectasia. The fact that these red spots are caused by telangiectasia can be demonstrated by pressing a glass slide on the lesions, which blanch on pressure. Such lesions can be found throughout the gastrointestinal tract and are the source of constant low-grade bleeding. The result is usually long-standing iron-deficiency anaemia, which responds to iron therapy. Occasionally larger, bleeding lesions may be found on endoscopy; these are amenable to local injection. Similar lesions are found in the nasal mucosa, and another common presentation is recurrent epistaxis. Once again, an individual lesion may be identified as being actively bleeding. In the nose there is some evidence that systemic oestrogen therapy may be of value. Lesions may also be found at other sites, especially the urogenital tract and the lung,

ANSWERS

where they may be associated with large numbers of AV malformations. The disease is transmitted as a dominant gene and multiple members of a family are usually affected. Genetic counselling should be given but may not be heeded. In the past, many patients were treated with blood transfusion to correct anaemia, with the result that many developed hepatitis and chronic liver disease, which compounded the bleeding problem. In addition, there is in some patients a deficiency of factor VIII (von Willebrand's factor), and levels may be low enough to have haemostatic implications.

74. This is a gouty tophus and is a reflection of the patient's long-standing hyperuricaemia. He has had multiple episodes of acute joint disease, particularly affecting the metatarso-phalangeal joints of the great toes. Needle aspiration of the tophus and microscopic examination of the aspirate shows multiple needle-shaped crystals of monosodium urate, which are negatively birefringent on polarized light microscopy. Treatment is with long-term allopurinol.

75. This man has chronic iron-deficiency anaemia. He has obvious pallor of the skin and mucous membranes. The dominant additional feature is the marked spooning (koilonychia) of his finger nails; the curvature of the nail is altered to such an extent that a drop of water can often be balanced on the convex surface of the nail. There may be other evidence of iron deficiency, in particular angular stomatitis, smoothness of the mucosa of the tongue and, sometimes, difficulty in swallowing due to an oesophageal web (Paterson-Brown-Kelly or Plummer-Vinson syndrome). Investigations should be directed towards finding the cause of the iron deficiency, which is usually long standing and may be related to insufficient dietary intake of iron as well as to chronic blood loss. Note that this man was also a heavy smoker, as shown by the tar staining of the index and middle fingers of the right hand.

76. This man has a left lower motor neurone lesion of the left 12th (hypoglossal) nerve. The hypoglossal nerve is wholly motor, supplying the tongue and the depressors of the hyoid. When the tongue is protruded the paralysis and wasting results in the tongue being pushed over to the paralysed side, as shown in this picture. Fasiculation may often be seen from the early stages of this nerve lesion.

77. There is distension of the external jugular vein up to the angle of the jaw, suggesting an elevated jugular venous pressure (JVP). It is important when examining neck veins that the patient is properly positioned in bed, lying at 45° to the horizontal. Check that the elevation of the JVP is bilateral and independent of neck rotation, to exclude the possibility that it may be the result of local constriction of the vein. Examine the patient for other signs of cardiac failure. This patient was clearly in congestive cardiac failure with peripheral oedema of the legs and sacrum, ascites and a right-sided hydrothorax. Assess the form of the venous pulse; it showed two peaks in this patient, confirming that she was in sinus rhythm. On gentle compression of the abdomen the distension of the vein increased (the hepatojugular reflux).

78. This man has abdominal distension associated with a line of indentation where the elasticated top of his trousers has applied pressure to the skin. In addition there are some superficial venous flares on the abdominal skin. His abdomen had been swelling for the past month, in association with a loss of appetite and intermittent nausea. Examination of the abdomen showed it to be tightly distended and no organs or masses could be felt. Percussion showed a large amount of gas with shifting dullness. The diagnosis proved to be carcinoma of the colon, with peritoneal metastases and hepatomegaly due to hepatic metastases.

79. This woman has neurofibromatosis (von Recklinghausen's disease). This is a rare disorder that is transmitted as an autosomal dominant. She has multiple neurofibromas and over the years several had been biopsied as they were increasing in size. In this view there are no apparent café-au-lait spots (the other characteristic skin feature of the disorder) but she did have freckling in her axillae, and was eventually shown to have a phaeochromocytoma which accounted for her intermittent hypertension. Neurofibromatosis occurs in two distinct types. This woman had Type I disease, which is due to an abnormality in chromosome 17, and is generally associated with predominantly peripheral lesions. Type II disease is generally associated with central lesions, such as acoustic neuromas and meningiomas. It results from an abnormality on chromosome 22. Antenatal diagnosis using gene markers is possible, and all such patients require counselling.

80. This man was diagnosed as having systemic sclerosis a year before this picture was taken. He had a long history of Raynaud's phenomenon, but the hand was generally warm except in the areas of obvious gangrenous changes. The skin of the fingers appeared slightly thickened and tight. No telangiectasia are apparent on this view, and there was no involvement of the mouth or oesophagus. The ESR was raised to 60mm in the first hour and he had a normochromic normocytic anaemia. The RA latex test was positive and anti-nuclear antibodies were present. The anti-scl70 and the anti-centromere antibody were negative. As can be seen by the tar staining of this man's thumb he is still smoking, and this should be actively discouraged. Raynaud's phenomenon may respond to simple measures such as the use of heated gloves, and calcium antagonists may also be of value. The prognosis for this type of systemic sclerosis is reasonably good provided the patients complies with medical advice.

81. This lady has an upper motor neurone lesion of the right facial nerve (nerve VII) of acute onset. Even at rest this is apparent and there is some difference between the nasolabial fold on the right hand side and the left. When she smiles, there is weakness of the muscles in the lower part of the face, especially around the mouth and eyes. As the forehead is bilaterally innervated, wrinkling of the brow remains obvious on both sides (in contrast to the asymmetry that occurs in lower motor neurone lesions, e.g. Bell's palsy). Examination showed a left carotid artery bruit and a Doppler ultrasound scan of the neck showed a stenosis of the left carotid artery. CT scan confirmed the presence of a thrombotic stroke. Immediate treatment of this patient was with aspirin but she should also be further evaluated for possible carotid artery surgery, the success of which is largely dependent on the degree of carotid artery stenosis.

82. The straight *x*-ray of the abdomen taken in the supine position shows colonic dilatation (toxic megacolon). This complication usually presents acutely with a tender swollen abdomen that is tympanitic due to the amount of gas which is in the colon. The patient was in shock, with a tachycardia and falling blood pressure, temperature was elevated and the abdomen was silent on auscultation. The leucocyte count was markedly elevated. This complication requires intensive management, with the replacement of fluids to sustain hydration and blood pressure, intravenous steroids and combination therapy with antibiotics. If the patient does not settle rapidly, surgery should be considered, due to the high risk of colonic perforation associated with peritonitis.

83. This patient has multiple vesicular lesions that have an erythematous base on the glans and shaft of his penis. These were accompanied by a low-grade fever, malaise and bilateral, tender inguinal adenopathy. Many of the lesions rapidly proceeded to ulceration and had a greyish-white exudate at the base of the ulcer. Healing occurred within two weeks. The lesions are typical of genital herpes simplex. It is important in such patients to enquire about sexual partners, and treatment should be offered to them as well. It is also important to remind staff that herpes simplex lesions are extremely infectious. Idoxuridine and acyclovir are indicated for the treatment of genital herpes.

84. The characteristic features here are periorbital oedema, which has caused the eyes to close, and gross facial oedema. If these changes were of acute onset, they could represent angioedema (e.g. resulting from an allergic reaction to a bee or wasp sting) but this 20-year-old man had been ill for the past six weeks with heavy proteinuria, hypoalbuminaemia and progressive generalized oedema, especially of the face. He has severe nephrotic syndrome. Causes of nephrotic syndrome include glomerulonephritis, diabetes mellitus, amyloidosis, multi-system disease such as SLE, neoplasia, infection and drug therapy such as gold, penicillamine and captopril. The cause of the disease is often not immediately obvious and renal biopsy is usually required in adults to establish a diagnosis and prognosis (membranous glomerulonephritis in this patient). Treatment depends on renal function and may include fluid and dietary sodium restriction, high protein intake and the judicious use of diuretics. Infusions of albumin may be of temporary value. Corticosteroid treatment is valuable in minimal-change glomerular lesions and may often be used without renal biopsy in children, where steroid-responsive minimal- change glomerular lesions are the usual underlying cause. In adults they should only be used after biopsy confirmation of a steroid-responsive disorder.

85. This is the mite *Sarcoptes scabiei* (variant *hominis*). Transmission of this disease is by close body contact and it is most commonly seen in times of war, poor housing and social unrest. The adult mite burrows in the skin and lays eggs resulting in the typical clinical appearances. A lesion may be probed with a sterile needle and the contents examined under the microscope to make a definite diagnosis. The common clinical feature is severe itching, usually more prominent at night time, and there may be secondary eczema. To prevent spread in the family, bedclothes and clothes should be thoroughly disinfested, and the entire family or other close contacts should be examined and treated if necessary.

86. This man has cardiomegaly with a cardiothoracic ratio of 54 per cent. In addition there are bilateral pleural effusions, with shadowing suggesting bilateral alveolar oedema. There is also probably a small pericardial effusion but this is best detected by echocardiography. This patient had congestive cardiac failure with peripheral oedema, sacral oedema, ascites and jugular venous congestion. The underlying diagnosis was ischaemic heart disease. Active treatment with diuretics led to rapid resolution of the appearances on the x-ray.

87. This woman was shorter – 5ft (1.52m) – and smaller than any other member of her family, which suggests that her problem had existed since childhood. She was also very thin – 88lbs (40kg) – and had poorly developed secondary sexual characteristics. Malabsorption was confirmed biochemically, and she had a mixed anaemia, with both iron and folate deficiency. The diagnosis of coeliac disease was confirmed by a small bowel biopsy. A gluten-free diet relieved her steatorrhoea and she gained weight. She should be maintained on a gluten-free diet for life and may require supplemental vitamins and minerals. It is important to keep such patients under review in the long term, as there is a significant incidence of small-intestinal lymphoma. Extra-gastrointestinal cancers and intestinal carcinoma are also more common in these patients.

88. This young man has acne vulgaris on his chest (also present on his face), which is an extremely common disorder in post-pubertal males and females. It is probably due to increased sebum production associated with infection of the pilo-sebaceous unit by *Propionibacterium acnes*. The generalized abnormality underlying the increased end-organ sensitivity within the sebaceous gland is a fluctuation in the androgen:oestrogen ratio. As can be seen there are a range of lesions on the chest from small papules and pustules to comedones and large painful cysts, all on a background of seborrhoea. Some of the healing scars have over grown, producing a keloid.

89. This is a double-contrast barium enema. The patient presented with recurrent attacks of diarrhoea that were usually bloodstained. The barium enema confirms the presence of active ulcerative colitis, with a fine nodular appearance and ulceration throughout the colon. There is also a loss of the normal haustrations, especially in the sigmoid and ascending colon. The barium has entered the terminal ileum, and fine granular ulceration is also clearly seen there (so-called backwash ileitis). The diagnosis was confirmed by colonoscopy with biopsy, and treatment with steroids and mesalazine instituted.

90. This patient has a healing ulcer of the skin of the shaft of the penis and ulceration in the pubic region and groin, which is partly concealed by his pubic hair. The diagnosis is likely to be a sexually transmitted disease. Chancroid, granuloma inguinale and lymphogranuloma venereum may all be associated with this range of features. This patient had lymphogranuloma venereum. This is caused by *Chlamydia trachomatis* and is most commonly found in tropical countries. The primary ulcerative lesion appears soon after sexual contact and is usually on the genitalia, but may also be found in the anus or on the lips and mouth; this heals rapidly but is followed by regional lymph node enlargement. The lymph nodes undergo suppuration and the pus discharges through the skin. In addition, there is generalized systemic upset with pyrexia, joint involvement, splenomegaly and occasionally meningism. Healing may leave extensive scarring with stricture of the vagina, urethra or rectum. Treatment is with tetracycline. The suppurating lymph nodes should be aspirated to prevent sinus formation.

91. This view shows proliferative retinopathy with extensive formation of new vessels in several areas. In addition, there is vitreous haemorrhage and numerous areas of photocoagulation with typical, circular black scars. The patient has long-standing insulin-dependent dia

ANSWERS

betes and has been under the care of an ophthalmologist for some years, due to progressive visual impairment. This is the only likely cause of this fundal appearance, reinforcing the need for tight control of the diabetic state, in order to postpone such complications.

92. This patient has developed acute surgical emphysema following the pneumothorax or its treatment. His face has doubled in size, and on palpation of his skin, the typical feel of air in the subcutaneous tissues was present all over his head, neck and chest wall. Surgical emphysema is usually of trivial importance but may occasionally be life-threatening due to compression of vital structures. On this occasion the air resorbed with no specific treatment and the pneumothorax resolved after removal and repositioning of the intrapleural catheter.

93. This patient's hand shows a generalized but patchy increase in pigmentation and multiple ulcers, which may have resulted from the breakdown of blistering lesions. Note the tar staining of his index finger – a sure sign of heavy smoking. These are the changes seen in variegate porphyria and porphyria cutanea tarda. The presence of excess porphyrins in the circulation leads to photosensitivity of exposed areas with local blister formation and the formation of pigmented scars. In addition, there is abnormal mechanical fragility of the skin. In this patient porphyria cutanea tarda was associated with chronic liver disease and long-term excessive intake of alcohol. The disease is caused by an inherited deficiency of uroporphyrinogen decarboxylase and as a result there may be an increased excretion of uroporphyrin, which may give the urine a pink-brown colouration. It is important for these patients to avoid alcohol and to protect their skin from sunlight.

94. The red cells have sedimented almost totally within 20 minutes to form a packed cell layer that is only about 30 per cent of the total volume, indicating that the patient is anaemic and has a very high sedimentation rate. The dominant feature is the size of the buffy coat which is massively elevated, indicating a very high white cell count. Above the buffy coat can be seen the outline of the small fibrin clot which formed after the cells sedimented. The small size of the fibrin clot is a reflection of the disseminated intravascular coagulation that was present. The absolute and differential white cell count will point to the diagnosis; in this case it proved to be chronic myeloid leukaemia.

95. This patient has been started on chronic ambulatory peritoneal dialysis (CAPD), carried out via a Tenckhoff peritoneal dialysis catheter. The intraperitoneal pressure rise during dialysis has resulted in the appearance of an umbilical hernia that is fluid filled.

96. This man was Caucasian, so the degree of skin pigmentation is clearly abnormal. It had developed over the preceding few years. This suggests a diagnosis of haemochromatosis (bronze diabetes). In this condition excessive iron is absorbed and deposited in internal organs, especially the liver, spleen, pancreas, pituitary and heart. Pigmentation of the skin is also found; this may be a slatey grey colour, but occasionally it becomes much browner due to the stimulation of melanocytes in the skin. Deposition of iron in the pancreas leads to deficiency in endocrine function and a reduction in insulin production, so that many patients become glucose intolerant or frankly diabetic. This patient had also suffered from joint pains over the last year, particularly in the knees, hips and small joints of the hands. These resulted from pyrophosphate arthropathy, with chondrocalcinosis. There was no evidence of cardiac involvement and his ECG was normal. Routine liver function tests showed changes consistent with early cirrhosis, but the liver was not palpable and the patient declined liver biopsy. Haemochromatosis is an inherited disease, and it is important that other family members are screened. One brother of this patient died of liver cirrhosis, but no postmortem was carried out and the diagnosis never fully confirmed. All family members were examined and the levels of serum iron, iron saturation, TIBC and ferritin measured. This patient was treated with long-term, repeated venesection.

97. This is aphthous ulceration. The painful lesions are common; typically a central ulcer surrounded by an erythematous border, which heals over one or two weeks.

Aphthous ulceration is usually an isolated problem of unknown cause, but severe ulceration may be associated with:

> Behçet's syndrome (usually multiple ulcers, found in association with genital ulceration and inflammatory ocular lesions).
>
> Gastrointestinal disease (i.e. coeliac disease, inflammatory bowel disease).
>
> AIDS

It is also important to exclude the possibility of malignant disease. Any ulcer in the oral cavity which fails to heal in two weeks should be considered as a potential squamous cell carcinoma. Malignant ulcers are usually painless and often arise in areas of pre-existing leukoplakia. Ulceration in association with gingival hyperplasia is seen in acute leukaemia.

98. There is a deep penetrating ulcer over the metatarsal head of the first toe of the left foot. The ulcer is well demarcated, with thickening of the surrounding skin. The second and third toes have been amputated. The site of the ulcer, on one of the pressure points of the feet, the surrounding thickened skin and the clean, well demarcated ulcer itself are typical of a neuropathic ulcer, and the likely underlying cause is diabetes mellitus.

99. The likely diagnosis is giant cell (temporal or cranial) arteritis. Premonitory symptoms may have included headache or scalp tenderness, jaw claudication, fever, weight loss, pain or stiffness in the shoulder or pelvic girdle muscles (features of polymyalgia rheumatica). The diagnosis is supported by a grossly elevated ESR and confirmed by temporal artery biopsy. The picture shows dilation of the right temporal artery which, in conjunction with sudden loss of vision, makes giant cell arteritis likely. Additional symptoms include those of polymyalgia rheumatica, which often coexists with giant cell arteritis. The diagnosis can only be confirmed by histological findings on temporal artery biopsy. However, due to the patchy distribution of the arteritis, negative histology should not prevent treatment, particularly if the ESR is elevated and a normochromic, normocytic anaemia is present.

100. This patient has a diffuse purpuric rash with larger areas of sheet haemorrhage (ecchymosis). These features, in association with the persistent infection, suggest marrow depression with thrombocytopenia and neutropenia. This was confirmed by the results of her full blood count, which showed a haemoglobin of 10.8g/dl, total white cell count of 2.8×10^9/l and platelets of 31×10^9/l. Bone marrow aspiration produced a dry tap at the sternum and marrow was only obtained by undertaking a trephine biopsy of her ilium.

The common causes include cytotoxic drugs, radiation, viruses, a wide range of other chemicals and drugs and leukaemic syndromes. The actual cause was never identified but one month prior to this presentation while on holiday in Spain she had purchased an antibiotic, which may have been chloramphenicol, from a local chemist.

101. There is wasting of the dorsal interossei and muscles of the thenar eminence. The causes of wasting of the small muscles of the hand include motor neurone disease, syringomyelia, meningovascular syphilis, tumour or trauma at T1 cord level or in the brachial plexus, cervical spondylosis, cord compression, ulnar or median nerve lesions and disuse atrophy due to arthritis. The absence of sensory changes and arthritis makes motor neurone disease the likely diagnosis in a middle-aged man.

102. The major finding is the presence of multiple calcified pleural plaques, which are strongly suggestive of asbestos-induced disease. The patient had worked with asbestos as a pipe lagger in the shipyards. He had also been a moderately heavy smoker and continued to smoke. There is no evidence of fibrotic changes in the lungs, and no asbestos bodies were found in his sputum, so he did not seem to have pulmonary asbestosis. Nevertheless, the combination of cigarette smoking and asbestos exposure have a synergistic action in promoting the subsequent onset of bronchial carcinoma. He is also at risk of pleural mesothelioma. Even at this stage, he should be encouraged to stop smoking.

103. The striking feature in 103a is bilateral ptosis, and this has been relieved in 103b. The underlying diagnosis is myasthenia gravis, and intravenous edrophonium chloride has been administered in the period between the two pictures being taken.

Edrophonium chloride is an anticholinesterase drug of very rapid onset but brief duration of action (approximately five minutes). It is used as a diagnostic test for myasthenia gravis by administering 2mg intravenously initially, followed by a further 8mg if no adverse reactions occur; typically it produces a rapid, short-lived alleviation of myasthenic symptoms as shown here. Cholinergic reactions can be reversed by intravenous atropine.

104. This woman has quite a marked buffalo hump, which is a pad of fat between the scapulae. She also exhibits hirsutism, with hair growth in "sideburn" distribution on the face, and over the buffalo hump itself. CT scan showed a pituitary tumour. The patient therefore has Cushing's disease, with a pituitary adenoma secreting excess ACTH and producing bilateral adrenal hyperplasia.

105. The optic disc is very pale, but it is flat (in focus throughout) and has a well-defined margin. The patient has optic atrophy of the "primary" type; this results from compression of the optic pathways by the pituitary tumour, rather than from long-term papilloedema.

106. This is an endoscopic retrograde cholangiopancreatogram (ERCP) showing gallstones in a dilated common bile duct. The intrahepatic ducts are not dilated. The patient might present with abdominal pain (acute pancreatitis or cholecystitis), obstructive jaundice, or with a fever and the systemic features of ascending cholangitis.

107. These are conjunctival haemorrhages, and the patient also has a corneal arcus. Conjunctival haemorrhages may be a manifestation of septic emboli or of immune complex vasculitis in infective endocarditis, the most likely explanation of this man's condition. His abdominal pain may result from splenic infarction. It is essential to confirm the diagnosis of infective endocarditis by blood culture and serology, and to establish the nature of the underlying cardiac disorder. The corneal arcus is probably an incidental finding.

108. This radiograph shows extensive pancreatic calcification, which is usually a sign of chronic pancreatitis. In the developed world, alcoholic pancreatitis is the usual problem; in the developing world, pancreatic calcification is commonly associated with non-alcoholic malnutrition-associated chronic pancreatitis.

109. The blue appearance of the patient's hand is caused by methaemoglobinaemia, a recognized side effect of therapy with dapsone. The skin rash for which he received the drug was dermatitis herpetiformis. This was associated with a gluten enteropathy similar to that of coeliac disease, for which he was recommended a gluten-free diet.

110. This is a typical left peritonsillar abscess (quinsy). It is likely to be caused by *Streptococcus pyogenes*, and should be treated with penicillin and surgical drainage or tonsillectomy if it proves to be unresponsive to antibiotic treatment alone. Note also the coated tongue and the presence of an exudate on the other tonsil.

111. This is a double-contrast barium meal, which shows a central ulcer crater in the duodenal cap. This is the typical appearance of a duodenal ulcer with barium filling the crater. There has been some scarring of the surrounding tissue, with drawing-in of the mucosal folds, which gives the radiating appearance of the barium. Such a patient should be investigated by endoscopy and antral biopsy. The biopsy samples can be tested for urease (a positive result suggests the presence of *Helicobacter pylori*), and cultured for *Helicobacter pylori*. Treatment should be instituted with an H_2 blocker or a proton pump inhibitor. If *Helicobacter pylori* are found, then "triple therapy" with bismuth, amoxycillin and metronizadole should be instigated, although other regimens (e.g. omeprazole plus amoxycillin) are also under investigation.

112. This is Fournier's gangrene of the penile shaft. The most common causative organism is a *Bacteroides* species (usually *B. fragilis*), which is an anaerobic gram-negative bacillus found in the human bowel. Antibiotics, debridement and later plastic surgery are necessary. The usual antibiotic given is metronidazole. The abdominal wall, perineum and thighs may also be involved.

113. This lesion is acanthosis nigricans, a dark brown or black, hyperpigmented, raised area of the skin that is smooth and velvety to the touch and may be found in the axillae, groin and around the umbilicus. Acanthosis nigricans may occur in some obese patients, particularly in association with insulin resistance syndromes. It may also occur in partial lipodystrophy, Cushing's syndrome and the Stein-Leventhal syndrome. Most commonly it is a skin manifestation of internal malignancy, particularly of adenocarcinoma of the stomach (60 per cent of cases), a diagnosis which is strongly suggested by this patient's other features.

114. The key features of the film are the presence of numerous Howell-Jolly bodies and punctate basophilia in the red cells. The red cells show anisocytosis and poikilocytosis with

ANSWERS

abnormal burr forms. There is thrombocytosis. This is the typical blood film of a person with splenic absence or hypofunction. It is typical of someone whose spleen has been removed surgically, usually for trauma; in addition, the possibility of congenital splenic absence, sickle cell disease or coeliac disease should be considered (though there are no features suggestive of sickle cell disease in this film). Patients with impaired or absent splenic function are at risk of overwhelming infection, especially with *Streptococcus pneumoniae*. They should be given appropriate advice and pneumococcal immunization. In addition, at times of stress or other infection the use of prophylactic antibiotics should be considered.

115. This patient shows wasting of the muscles of the upper leg, and signs of extreme weight loss, with prominent pelvic bones. There is a rash over the back, buttocks and upper legs. The likely cause of these findings is zinc deficiency, which may also cause alopecia, night blindness and ageusia. Zinc is a trace element essential for wound healing, enzyme activity and defence against infections. In severe Crohn's disease, there are significant intestinal fluid and mineral losses, resulting in zinc deficiency and the characteristic rash, which is often complicated by superficial staphylococcal and yeast infections. Treatment is by supplementation of the parenteral nutrition with zinc salts.

116. This woman is hyperpigmented and, in the light of her clinical history, Addison's disease (adrenocortical insufficiency) is the likely diagnosis. This can be confirmed by measuring the cortisol response to the intravenous or intramuscular injection of synthetic ACTH (Synacthen), in the short Synacthen test. The cause of her adrenal insufficiency was not established, but she had a strong family history of organ-specific autoimmune disorders.

117. The patient has severe left-sided facial weakness, resulting from lower motor neuron palsy of the seventh cranial (facial) nerve (see also answer 81, page 110). This is a classic example of Bell's palsy. The cause is probably usually viral, but is often unknown. The disease is usually self-limiting, and 90 per cent of patients achieve full recovery of facial nerve function.

118. This is an M-mode echocardiogram accompanied by a two-dimensional picture, which shows that it was recorded in the parasternal long-axis view. There is asymmetrical hypertrophy of the intraventricular septum (the thick band towards the top of the M-mode trace). The appearances are suggestive of hypertrophic obstructive cardiomyopathy (HOCM).

119. This patient has marked truncal obesity, with pink striae over the thorax and abdomen. Pink striae are common in obese individuals, who may also fail to suppress cortisol during an overnight dexamethasone suppression test. The normal cortisol response to hypoglycaemia differentiates simple obesity with failure of suppression of cortisol by dexamethasone from Cushing's syndrome. This boy had simple obesity.

120. This is the same patient's hand before and immediately after an "ice-water" immersion test. The technique used is thermography, which is a method of displaying infra-red radiation from the skin. The patient had a history of severe Raynaud's phenomenon. The left-hand picture was taken at a room temperature of 22°C, and blood flow was adequate in

120

the patient's hand at that time, as evidenced by the full image of the hand and its colour (note the colour/temperature scale to the right of the picture). The provocative test was to immerse the hand for two minutes in ice-water, and the result is shown in the right-hand picture, in which the dominant colours are blue and purple; the circulation to the distal part of the digits has totally disappeared. This is a very abnormal reaction which confirms vasospastic disease. Such patients must keep their hands warm and avoid sudden temperature changes. Heated gloves are helpful. Some patients require prophylactic treatment with a vasodilator such as nifedipine or other calcium channel blockers. In severe disease, permanent skin and subcutaneous tissue changes develop and digital gangrene may occur.

121. This very advanced lesion has a rolled, pearly edge in some parts and has eroded deeply into the subcutaneous tissues. Biopsy confirmed the clinical suspicion that this was an advanced basal cell carcinoma (rodent ulcer). Treatment is with radiotherapy and plastic surgery for reconstruction of the patient's nose and cheek. It is now rare to see such advanced disease in Western society. Early lesions can usually be treated by cryotherapy, radiotherapy and/or minor surgery.

122. The close-up of the palm shows a typical papulo-squamous rash (syphilide), which is the generalized form of secondary syphilis. The secondary stage follows the primary stage after a period of about two months and its other features include fever, snail-track ulcers in the buccal mucosa, generalized lymphadenopathy and occasionally aseptic meningitis. The condition is often self-limiting, and after a period of a few weeks symptoms may totally disappear, to be followed by a latent period apparently free of disease, which may range from two to 20 years, before the tertiary stages appear. The spirochaetes may be found in exudates during this secondary stage; serological tests such as the non-specific VDRL or an antitreponemal test (TPI, TPHA or FTA) should be carried out. Treatment is urgently required and should be given with a long-acting penicillin over a 14-day period. Steroids may also be used to prevent the Jarisch-Herxheimer reaction, which may otherwise develop as the spirochaetes die.

123. This is an ultrasound scan of the liver. It shows at least two nodular abnormalities representing metastases. The patient had a known primary carcinoma of the colon. The presence of liver metastases is most simply and non-invasively demonstrated by ultrasound, and the result has a major influence on future therapy.

124. This man has clearly lost weight, the sclerae and skin are yellow, and the finger he is using to pull down his right eyelid is tar-stained. He has obstructive jaundice due to metastatic bronchial carcinoma, which is the result of long-term cigarette smoking. Palliative care was all that was possible for him.

125. This patient has lupus pernio, which is part of the spectrum of chronic sarcoidosis. The term is used to describe the dusky purple infiltration of the skin of the nose, which is a relatively rare manifestation of sarcoidosis. This lady had no other skin involvement, but an x-ray of her chest showed bilateral hilar lymphadenopathy and pulmonary infiltration, which had been asymptomatic. She had also had painful swelling of the proximal interphalangeal joints of two of her fingers (dactylitis). The diagnosis of sarcoidosis may be made by biopsy

ANSWERS

of skin, lung or lymph nodes. The Mantoux test in this patient was negative but the Kveim test was not carried out. In this patient the level of the angiotensin-converting enzyme was raised and this was used to follow the progression of the disease. While minor involvement of skin or lymph nodes (including the hilar nodes) may be watched over a period of time without treatment (spontaneous resolution often occurs), the presence of lung lesions requires the administration of corticosteroids. Lupus pernio must be distinguished from the red nose often associated with chronic alcoholism, and from rhinophyma and acne rosacea.

126. This patient had psoriatic arthritis, which had been diagnosed several years previously and treated when necessary with non-steroidal anti-inflammatory drugs. However, in the preceding month he had had severe pain in the small joints of the toes, particularly in the interphalangeal joints, and had been aware of nodules that discharged a white material. This was associated with a flare-up of his skin psoriasis. Examination of the discharge under polarised light showed negative birefringent, needle-shaped crystals, confirming that the diagnosis was acute gout supervening in a patient with psoriasis and psoriatic arthropathy. Once the acute joint problem had settled with non-steroidal treatment the patient was started on allopurinol. Extensive psoriasis in exacerbation is associated with increased DNA turnover and excess urate production.

127. This man has a patchy, raised depigmented rash with a butterfly distribution over his cheeks and the bridge of the nose. In combination with polyarthritis, this suggests a diagnosis of systemic lupus erythematosus (SLE). SLE is relatively rare in men, but relatively common in patients of Afro-Caribbean origin. Routine examination of this patient's blood showed that he had leucopenia and thrombocytopenia. His ESR was raised at 90mm in the first hour and his plasma viscosity was high. The antinuclear antibody test was positive, confirming the diagnosis of SLE.

128. This patient has opaque white nails (leukonychia). These are found in a variety of conditions in which the serum albumin is low, including nephrotic syndrome and chronic liver disease. The patient had other stigmata of liver function impairment and was known to be a chronic alcoholic.

129. These are spider naevi. The typical raised central punctum is the point at which the spiral artery comes to the surface of the dermis. Radiating from this are the "legs" of the spider. Compression of the spiral artery by the head of a pin, or of the whole lesion with a glass slide, results in blanching of the whole lesion. When pressure is released, the lesion refills with blood from the centre. Such spider naevi are usually distributed in the territory drained by the superior vena cava and within this area are more commonly found in the light-exposed regions, e.g. the backs of the hands and forearms, the "V" of the neck and the face. They may be found in normal individuals but more than two or three should be considered abnormal, although they may appear in women physiologically – at the menarche and during pregnancy. Pathologically they are most common in patients with impaired liver function, probably as a result of defective metabolism of oestrogen. They may also be found in patients who are taking therapeutic oestrogens, e.g. for carcinoma of the prostate and in women taking oral contraceptives. They have been reported in a few patients with thyrotoxicosis and rheumatoid arthritis.

130. The DTPA scan (on the right) outlines the kidneys, because DTPA is excreted by glomerular filtration. MIBG is selectively taken up by tissues with sympathetic activity. This MIBG scan shows the uptake of a large amount of radionuclide on the patient's right, suggesting the presence of a phaechromocytoma. The renal outlines, shown in the DTPA scan, can be superimposed to localize the tumour to the right adrenal. Large tumours may also be easily identified on CT scan but the advantage of this radionuclide functional imaging technique is that it will pick up small tumours that may be present in organs other than adrenal, e.g. in the sympathetic chain.

131. This man has pre-existing chronic ischaemic changes in his leg, with atrophy of the muscles and skin pigmentation. The new feature is thrombophlebitis which extends up the leg. In the picture this is shown as an area of redness following the line of the superficial veins. This man subsequently developed other areas of migrating thrombophlebitis, and was eventually shown to have carcinoma of the pancreas (the commonest occult cause of migrating thrombophlebitis).

132. There are several areas of bruising in the abdominal wall; closer inspection of these shows a punctum in the centre. This is now a common feature in patients in most surgical and medical wards and is due to the use of subcutaneous low-dose heparin for thromboprophylaxis. The bruises occur only at the injection sites of these low doses of heparin. Occasionally the bruises may be raised if there is a reaction to the injection. Skin necrosis has been reported as a sequel to heparin injection. This can be prevented by the use of the abdominal wall as the injection site, and by a specific, careful injection technique designed to avoid damaging the skin and subcutaneous fat.

133. This 54-year-old man was admitted with an acute thrombotic stroke that has left him with a left-sided facial weakness. The second dominant feature is his high colour, which is due to polycythemia (primary proliferative polycythemia: PPP). Patients with a high haematocrit have an enhanced risk of thrombotic episodes. Thrombosis may be venous or arterial. The diagnosis of polycythaemia is suggested by the Coulter counter printout, in which the haemoglobin, haematocrit and red cell count are elevated, as may be the platelet count and white cell count. Confirmation of the diagnosis requires the measurement of plasma and red cell volume. Treatment is with repeated venesection.

134. The appearances are those of a left-sided pneumothorax. The edge of the left lung is best seen if followed upwards from the diaphragm. There is a small pleural reaction with fluid on the left, and fluid can also be seen in the left interlobar fissure. There is some tenting of the diaphragm on the left, which may be due to old adhesion. The patient was a tall, thin athletic male, but he did not satisfy the clinical criteria for Marfan's syndrome. As he was clinically stable and not dyspnoeic, a decision was made to allow the air to absorb spontaneously. There has been no recurrence to date of the lesion, which was presumed due to the spontaneous rupture of a bleb on the lung surface.

135. This lady has osteoarthritis with Heberden's nodes at the distal interphalangeal joint and Bouchard's nodes at the proximal interphalangeal joint. In addition, there is some fixed deformity with limitation of movement of the interphalangeal joints. Osteoarthritis is a common degenerative disease which affects approximately 10 per cent of all adults, the incidence and severity of the problem increasing with age. The cause is probably multifactorial although an early form may run within families. In addition, mechanical factors such as previous limb trauma, joint hyper-mobility and certain occupations may be relevant. Osteoarthritis is a complication of some metabolic disorders including ochronosis, acromegaly and gout. The symptoms suffered by this lady included stiffness after prolonged inactivity, some local pain and difficulty gripping objects. Clinical signs included crepitus, limitation of movement and joint deformity. In addition to the hands, her knees and hips were particularly affected. X-rays showed loss of joint space resulting from erosion of cartilage with osteophytes, altered bone contour, increased bone density and cyst formation. X-rays may also show tissue swelling in association with the joint abnormality and some periarticular calcification. Treatment is symptomatic pain relief with simple analgesics.

136. This echocardiogram shows a large apical thrombus in the left ventricle (LV) at the top of the picture. It is probable that the patient's hemiparesis is due to embolization of part of this thrombus to the cerebral vessels. Thrombus in the left ventricle most commonly follows acute myocardial infarction; several large studies show that about 30 per cent of patients with anterior myocardial infarction develop mural thrombi, and about 5 per cent of these mural thrombi throw off clinically significant emboli to the brain, kidneys or limbs. In this patient there was no clinical history to suggest myocardial infarction, but an ECG showed resolving changes of infarction, so it is likely that this was the original diagnosis. It is important to remember that if anterior myocardial infarction is diagnosed, prophylactic heparin (12,500 units b.d.) should be given to reduce the risk of mural thrombosis and embolism.

137. This man has cirrhosis of the liver of unknown aetiology. He recently developed extreme swelling of the abdomen, mainly due to ascites that has resulted from increasing portal hypertension and failing liver function. The collateral venous circulation is well illustrated over the surface of the abdomen and chest; the direction of blood flow was away from the umbilicus. The other obvious abnormality is the subcutaneous linear lesion running from the epigastrium to the neck. This is the line of a peritineo-venous shunt, which has been inserted to drain the ascitic fluid back into the circulation. These may sometimes be very effective in maintaining the plasma albumin level but may be a source of infection and obstruction.

138. The widespread petechiae and ecchymoses are typical of disseminated intravascular coagulation (DIC) associated with septicaemia. The most common cause is meningococcal septicaemia, but DIC may be found with other infections. This man clearly had acute septicaemia and had developed signs of meningism. Lumbar puncture and Gram staining of a slide of the CSF confirmed the diagnosis of meningococcal septicaemia. The was later confirmed by blood cultures. *Neisseria meningitides* is a Gram-negative diplococcus with a number of serotypes. Infection is transmitted by inhalation of droplets; the nose and pharynx are colonized, giving rise to a carrier state or disseminated infection. Meningococcal infection usually affects specific groups, including young children and adults in a closed environment such as an army camp or school. This patient's fulminating septicaemia was associated with the Waterhouse-Friderichsen syndrome, with DIC, extensive skin haemorrhages, and acute adrenal and circulatory failure. Often such patients do not live long enough to develop the full picture of meningitis. Antibiotic treatment should be started immediately with intravenous benzylpenicillin given in large doses. In addition, intensive nursing care is required and occasionally, in the severely affected patient with circulatory collapse, large doses of steroids may be required. Effective vaccines are available against Groups A and C meningococci and are indicated in high-risk situations.

139. This sputum sample, which is a rusty brown colour with a tinge of red, is from a patient with haemoptysis. The rusty brown colour is due to the degradation of the haemoglobin to hemosiderin. The patient developed an aspiration pneumonia after attempting suicide by jumping from the Tay Bridge. It was once considered that rusty sputum was pathognomonic of pneumonia but other causes of haemoptysis must always be considered, such as bronchial carcinoma, tuberculosis, pulmonary embolism, bronchiectasis and Goodpasture syndrome.

140. This chest x-ray shows total consolidation of the right lung. The 67-year-old male patient also had a permanent cardiac pacemaker in situ. He had been a life-long smoker and is known to have chronic obstructive airways disease. He had been drinking to excess since the death of his wife four years previously and had early evidence of hepatic dysfunction. He was admitted with fever of two days duration and had been complaining of right-sided pleuritic chest pain. He was initially diagnosed as having lobar pneumonia but his condition worsened despite therapy with amoxycillin. By the time of admission to hospital he had developed the features shown in the x-ray. He had evidence of multi-system disease with renal impairment, liver dysfunction and early encephalopathy. Blood culture was taken and therapy was started urgently with ciprofloxacin, the presumption being that he had Legionnaires' disease. Despite therapy he died on the second day after admission. Postmortem confirmed the extent of the pneumonic consolidation and culture eventually confirmed that it was due to *Legionella*. The risk of dying from this condition is increased by advancing years, male sex, cigarette smoking, alcohol excess and previous chronic chest disease or immunosuppression. The source of this man's infection was never found. The organism is widespread, but a search of his home environment, showerheads and taps was negative.

141. These lesions are circular plaques of scaling erythema. Their appearance, itchiness and circular shape suggest the possibility of ringworm, and the patient's occupation enhanced the possibility that this could be of animal origin. The diagnosis was confirmed by observing blue-green fluorescence under Wood's light and by microscopy and culture of skin scrapings. This infection was with *Trichophyton verrucosa*, which usually affects animals.

142. This young female has vulval herpes simplex causing severe local inflammation and ulceration. She also had local lymph node involvement bilaterally, the nodes being swollen and tender. Vaginal examination was impossible due to the intense pain. No herpes simplex lesions were found elsewhere. Treatment with acyclovir was required and because of the severity of the presentation this was started intravenously. In addition, local acyclovir cream was applied to the labia and vagina. The course of treatment is usually five days but in severely affected patients a longer course may be needed. As with all sexually transmitted disorders an attempt should be made to follow-up recent sexual partners, but this proved impossible in this situation, as the partner was a casual acquaintance in Greece.

143. This is a recurrence of bullous pemphigoid; on this occasion the blisters, which are large and tense, have occurred on the patient's leg, but they may affect any part of the skin surface. They are usually preceded by intense itching and may be associated with an eczematous eruption. The blisters are sub-epidermal in site and immunofluorescence shows linear IgG at the dermal/epidermal junction. By contrast, the blisters in pemphigus are intra-epidermal.

144. This x-ray shows multiple calcified foci, almost certainly due to old tuberculosis. Both upper zones are particularly affected and there is also calcification of the lymph nodes at both hila. There is no evidence of active disease and this is a common finding in patients born before 1940 in the UK. It is not a cause for concern before surgery unless this is to be followed by corticosteroid or other immunosuppressive therapy, which may lead to reactivation of the tuberculosis.

145. This man is likely to have dermatomyositis, with a typical presentation of discomfort and weakness of the girdle muscles of the shoulders and pelvis. The skin rash is typical. It usually affects the face and neck and often extends over the trunk and arms. A heliotrope rash may occur on the eyelids and is associated with telangiectasia in about 15 per cent of patients. Some patients also develop arthralgia and Raynaud's syndrome but these features were not present in this case. In this age group there is a common association with various types of malignancy, in particular with tumours of the stomach and lung in males and breast and ovary in females. Laboratory investigations of value include a profile of muscle enzyme levels; abnormalities may be found in the electromyogram; and muscle biopsy usually shows an inflammatory cell infiltration. In the acute phase, where there is muscle weakness or pain, bedrest is important and treatment may be given with high-dose corticosteroids and immunosuppressive drugs such as azathioprine, cyclophosphamide and methotrexate.

146. This is a barium meal which shows a large, fungating, space-occupying lesion in the fundus of the stomach. Endoscopic biopsy confirmed that this was a gastric carcinoma. The patient presented with weight loss and iron-deficiency anaemia due to alimentary blood loss. The only treatment which might be of value is surgery but the prognosis is poor, and before it is undertaken a careful search must be made for evidence of metastases. Liver metastases were found in this patient. Palliative surgery may occasionally be helpful, even when metastases are present, since such tumours are not readily amenable to chemotherapy or radiotherapy.

147. This is an M-mode echocardiogram of the aortic root. The two bright outer lines represent the aortic root and the box-like structure within these lines the aortic valve cusps. In systole, the cusps open, clearly suggesting that there is no aortic stenosis. The closure line is central, suggesting the valve has the normal complement of three cusps. A bicuspid aortic valve usually has an eccentric closure line. From the evidence shown here this aortic valve would be considered normal.

148.   This patient has alcaptonuria, which is a hereditary disorder caused by the absence of the enzyme homogentisic acid oxidase. The result of this defect is that homogentisic acid produced by degradation of phenylalanine and tyrosine cannot be further metabolized and therefore accumulates in the body. It is excreted in the urine and many patients present in childhood, due to the brown colour that develops in nappies (diapers). This is due to a reduction product of the colourless homogentisic acid. Homogentisic acid tends to pigment cartilage and other connective tissues including the sclera (ochronosis), and eventually causes a degenerative arthropathy, as seen in this patient's knees. The pathophysiology of the arthritis is unknown, and no prophylactic or curative treatment is available. Gene therapy may prove possible in the future.

149.   This female patient has extensive erysipelas over her forehead, cheeks and neck. This skin infection spreads through the tissue planes very rapidly. The infecting organism is *Streptococcus pyogenes.* The infected area is red, warm and sometimes quite tender. At the edge of the rash there is a well-demarcated, firm edge. The local lymph nodes are usually enlarged and tender. Penicillin is still the treatment of choice and the antibiotic therapy should be continued for seven to 10 days. Usually no site of entry for the organism is found.

150.   This 62-year-old male patient has multiple renal stones (nephrolithiasis), with a large "staghorn" calculus in the right kidney. He presented with attacks of recurrent urinary tract infection that had been treated intermittently with antibiotics by his family doctor. On this occasion he had bilateral colicky lumbar pain, which led to his being seen in hospital. He had spent much of his working life in the Middle East, which may have been of some aetiological significance. Examination of his urine showed that he had an infection with *E. coli*, and his renal function was impaired (elevation of the serum creatinine and reduction of creatinine clearance). Calculi of this size must usually be removed by open surgery. Smaller stones may be removed by percutaneous surgery, or their bulk may be reduced by this technique prior to treatment by lithotripsy. Small renal stones may often be treated by lithotripsy alone.

151.   This patient has bilateral multiple punched-out ulcers. As can be seen from the skin in his legs, these have been present before and have healed over with thin, atrophic skin, often associated with brown pigmentation due to hemosiderin deposition. The active ulcer base is very necrotic and is secondarily infected. The appearance is typical of vasculitic ulcers. The background disease in this patient is chronic rheumatoid arthritis, and this has symmetrically affected the small joints of both feet, which are swollen, tender, stiff and deformed. In addition to the vasculitic ulcers, this patient had other vasculitic lesions on his arm and subcutaneous rheumatoid nodules. There were no nail bed infarctions or splinter haemorrhages and he had no evidence of involvement of the sclerae. *X*-ray of the chest was normal. Immunological investigation showed a positive rheumatoid factor (a circulating immunoglobulin of the IgM type). In addition, teh patient had a normocytic normochromic anaemia with markedly elevated ESR (80mm in the first hour) and elevation of the white cell count at $19x10^9$/l. The patient is currently taking penicillamine.

152.   The first possibility is a basal cell carcinoma (rodent ulcer), but the edge is raised, it is quite red in colour, the base of the ulcer is necrotic, and the speed of growth is exceptional for a rodent ulcer. The second possibility is a squamous cell carcinoma, but again the speed of growth is against this. Histology of the biopsy showed the typical appearance of Hodgkin's disease with Reed-Sternberg cells, and the disease was found on chest x-ray in which hilar lymphadenopathy was present. This is an unusual cutaneous manifestation of Hodgkin's disease and other lymphomas but such lesions may occur, and similar appearances may result from secondaries of other tumours.

153. Use of infra-red photography highlights the subcutaneous veins. As shown here, there is a massive collateral circulation superficially on the chest wall, which results from superior vena caval (SVC) obstruction. The patient's presentation to his family doctor had been with swelling of the face, which was more marked in the morning and disappeared during the daytime. By the time this picture was taken he had permanent swelling of the head and neck with engorgement of the neck veins. In addition, engorgement of the retinal veins was a dominant feature on fundoscopy. The underlying diagnosis was carcinoma of the bronchus. This patient was treated with radiotherapy to the upper mediastinum, which relieved the SVC obstruction.

154. This is a thallium perfusion scan of the heart. Thallium 201 is a radionuclide that is taken up by the myocardium in a similar manner to the potassium ion, via the Na/K ATPase system. The isotope is injected via a peripheral vein and the images obtained with the gamma camera. At peak exercise the myocardial uptake is dependent on the myocardial blood flow and the viability of myocardial cells. In this case the inferior region does not take up thallium at peak exercise. If this perfusion defect is also present at rest the appearances suggest a previous myocardial infarction. If this area of myocardium takes up thallium at rest there is a reversible perfusion defect, which suggests myocardial ischaemia. The technique may be used to test the success of percutaneous transluminal coronary angioplasty (PTCA) or coronary artery by-pass grafting in establishing reperfusion of viable myocardium.

155. This patient has a marked corneal arcus, which may be a reflection of long-standing hypercholesterolaemia associated with the increased protein turnover of the nephrotic syndrome. These patients are susceptible to premature atheroma and arterial thrombosis. Dietary and drug control of the cholesterol level may be required in the long term. Premature corneal arcus may also be a familial abnormality of no serious consequence, so it is essential to measure blood lipids before initiating therapy.

156. There are multiple patchy areas of skin necrosis but the rest of the foot is pink and on palpation was warm to the touch. The peripheral pulses (dorsalis pedis and the posterior tibial) were both palpable. However, capillary return in the non-gangrenous digits was poor. The patient was a long-standing insulin-dependent diabetic whose control has been poor over many years. This picture shows typical diabetic gangrene due to small vessel disease. Treatment consists of tight diabetic control, infusion of a prostacyclin derivative, and antibi otic therapy, as these superficial necrotic lesions are often infected. Surgical intervention was eventually needed to remove gangrenous skin and to amputate the left great toe.

157. This man presented with massive lymph node enlargement in the submental, cervical and supraclavicular lymph nodes. The nodes were non-tender, discrete and mobile. His lower lip is enlarged, but this was a long-term appearance, associated with mental retardation. On questioning, he admitted to having night sweats over at least the past three months. General examination showed a spleen tip 3cm below the left costal margin but no other lymphadenopathy was found clinically. Chest x-ray showed bilateral hilar node involvement. Lymph node biopsy showed the typical appearances of Hodgkin's disease with a IVB grading. Other possible causes of such widespread lymph node enlargement include non-Hodgkin's lymphoma, chronic lymphatic leukaemia (mainly in elderly patients) and – occasionally – tuberculosis. Treatment was initiated with combination therapy including mustine, vincristine, procarbazine and prednisolone (MOPP).

158. This is a barium swallow showing achalasia of the cardia. It was carried out in a 68-year-old man who had complained of dysphagia and food retention in the lower oesophagus. He had been treated previously by his family doctor for pneumonia and it is possible that this resulted from aspiration from the dilated oesophagus. In achalasia, the lower oesophageal sphincter fails to relax and the impaired peristalsis results in oesophageal retention of food. The diagnosis can be confirmed by oesophageal manometry. It is important to differentiate this condition from oesophageal carcinoma and this may require oesophagoscopy and biopsy. Treatment is by dilatation or occasionally by cardiomyotomy.

159. This man has had a major bleed into subcutaneous tissues of the axilla, arm and chest wall. The site of bleeding may have been precipitated by the use of a crutch but, in addition, he had been taking non-prescribed tablets for discomfort in his knee. These tablets contained aspirin. A drug interaction is the commonest cause of failure of control of warfarin therapy. A combination of warfarin and aspirin is particularly liable to cause bleeding as the two drugs act on different parts of the haemostatic mechanism: aspirin affects platelets, while warfarin depresses the level of the liver production of factors II, VII, IX and X. Every patient on warfarin should be reminded to examine the contents of any "over the counter" medication and especially to avoid aspirin. As there was no evidence of any compression of vital structures (arteries or nerves) it was decided that the aspirin should be stopped and the level of warfarin significantly reduced to bring the INR to 2. Bleeding ceased and the appearance ultimately resolved. It is important to continue the warfarin because of the risk (one in 10) of fatal pulmonary embolism.

160. This is severe eczema herpeticum. Patients who have atopic dermatitis (eczema) have defective cell-mediated immunity and are generally more susceptible to bacterial, viral and fungal infections. This patient has developed a herpes simplex infection of the face and other areas of his body. The typical crusted lesions at different stages of evolution are present, and some of these are confluent and haemorrhagic. Treatment with acyclovir is urgently required.

161. This lady was known to have chronic oedema of both legs that was woody hard and non-pitting. This was ascribed to congenital abnormality of the lymphatics but had not been fully investigated. She presented with a painful and tender swollen foot and lower leg. This is due to spreading cellulitis in her already swollen leg. The cellulitis responded to a prolonged course of penicillin. The main differential diagnosis here was an acute venous thrombosis, but this rarely presents with such a florid appearance or with generalived symptoms: and ultrasound examination of the calf, popliteal and femoral veins was negative.

162. There is calcification along the entire length of the brachial artery and its branches. The rigid wall of the radial artery was palpable at the wrist, and the appearance was also found in the lower limb vessels. The patient had chronic renal failure and renal osteodystrophy.

163. There is swelling of the wrist, metacarpophalangeal and interphalangeal joints (particularly the proximal ones). In addition, there is "swan neck" deformity of the little finger and wasting of the interosseous muscles of both hands. The dominant joint affected is the metacarpophalangeal joint, which causes severe restriction of finger movement. This is the typical appearance of the hands of a patient who has the symmetrical polyarthritis of rheumatoid arthritis. The diagnosis in this patient was confirmed by serology.

164. In the centre of the slide are shown groups of blast cells that are hypergranular with oval or bi-lobed nuclei. Characteristically these cells contain multiple yellow-staining Auer rods, often arranged in bundles as shown here. Occasionally these abnormal cells may be broken up, leaving Auer rods free in the circulation or in the preparation. It is common for a 15/17 chromosome translocation to be present in the M3 variant. The diagnosis is acute myeloblastic leukaemia (hypergranular promyelocytic leukaemia M3 variant).

165. This woman has advanced carcinoma of the left breast. She had been aware of a bloodstained discharge from the nipple for the past 18 months, but had been too afraid to seek medical advice. As can be seen, there is an extensive, infiltrating lesion, which has destroyed the nipple area, and a satellite lesion further up in the breast, which is swollen and retracted. There is also superficial lymphoedema and a spreading cellulitic appearance on the chest wall. Lymph nodes were palpable in the left axilla. The patient has been prepared for radiotherapy, which will be given in association with the anti-oestrogen preparation tamoxifen.

166. This girl has tuberous sclerosis (epiloia) with typical facial lesions (adenoma sebaceum). Other features that should be looked for are fibromas of the nail bed, shagreen patches at the base of the spine, ash leaf patches (white oval patches on the thorax), and nodules in the retina (phakomas). In addition, routine x-ray of the skull may show calcification in the walls of the lateral ventricle and there is an association with intracranial gliomas and hamartoma of the kidney. This disease is transmitted as an autosomal dominant and is associated with mental retardation and epilepsy. Little can be done for the facial lesions but if not too numerous they may be amiable to cosmetic surgery. Genetic counselling is required because of the dominant nature of the transmission of the disease and control of epilepsy is essential.

167. This man has a swollen ankle joint that was exquisitely tender and warm with a large effusion. Note also the skin lesion above the left ankle and patchy erythematous lesions on his right leg. The differential diagnosis of the acutely inflamed joint includes septic arthritis, acute gout, rheumatoid arthritis and the connective tissue diseases associated with arthropathy. The diagnosis should be confirmed by joint aspiration with microscopy and culture of the aspirate. Often direct Gram staining of the film will give the answer. The clinical presentation of patients with septic arthritis is typical; usually a single joint is involved. The joint becomes red, warm and swollen, and has a demonstrable effusion. Infecting organisms may be staphylococci, pneumococci, gonococci or Gram-negative bacilli. Often the organism may be found not only in joint fluid at aspiration but also in the blood on culture. There is usually a source of infection elsewhere, and culture of other suspicious lesions or discharges is also required. This picture was taken at a sexually transmitted disease clinic, which the patient had attended for a purulent urethral discharge that had all the characteristics of gonorrhoea. Treatment of gonorrhoea is with a penicillin although a range of newer antibiotics may be used including spectinomycin, the cephalosporins and ciprofloxacin. Contact tracing is important in all sexually transmitted diseases.

168. This x-ray shows shadowing due to advanced pulmonary tuberculosis affecting the apices and mid-zones of both lungs. There is early cavitation, particularly in the lesions on the right, and bilateral hilar lymphadenopathy. Tuberculosis is still uncommon in the United Kingdom and most Western countries, although the incidence is increasing worldwide. It should be particularly suspected in immigrants, in the elderly and in those who have immunodeficiency of any cause, particularly those with HIV infection.

169. This is a smooth tongue due to the absence of the filiform papillae. It is often called a "raw beef" tongue and is seen in deficiency of vitamin B. This 55-year-old man presented to the neurologists with a one-month history of bilateral loss of sensation in the feet with some tingling and numbness. Clinical examination showed that he had posterior column features, in particular loss of sensation of the ankle joint, loss of vibration sense and loss of the ankle jerk. Examination of a peripheral blood film showed that he had a macrocytosis, and marrow examination confirmed megaloblastic change. The diagnosis was confirmed by the finding of a low serum B_{12} with a positive two-stage Schilling test. B_{12} deficiency usually presents with the symptomatology of anaemia but on this occasion with symmetrical paraesthesia of the hands and feet, and impairment of proprioception and vibration produced ataxia that brought the patient to the attention of the neurologist.

170. This man has rhinophyma. This is usually a long-term complication of acne rosacea in which there is hyperplasia of the sebaceous glands and connective tissue of the nose, resulting in this "strawberry-like" appearance. In addition the orifices of the follicles are enlarged and the general appearance is of a bright red or purple colour. There may be associated changes of acne rosacea but this is not evident in this view of the patient. The major differential diagnosis is sarcoidosis (lupus pernio) in which there is diffuse bluish purple plaque formation over the nose and the surrounding skin of the cheek.

171. This x-ray shows a knee joint replacement. Examination of the bones gives the clue to the original pathology: there is "squaring" of the lower end of the patella and considerable destruction of bone in the femoral condyles and the tibial head. New bone and cyst formation can be seen in these sites, and bone cysts can also be seen in the patella. The underlying disease is haemophilia, associated with repeated haemarthroses of the knee.

172. This child has gross apparent hypertrophy of the calf muscles. Despite this the muscles were weak on formal testing, and for the boy to rise from the prone position, he had to "walk" his hands and feet towards each other, then walk his hands up the front of his leg to reach the upright position. This is known as Gowers' sign and is typically found in patients with Duchenne muscular dystrophy. The diagnosis is usually obvious on the clinical features alone but measurement of the creatine kinase value showed it to be massively elevated. The electromyogram (EMG) and muscle biopsy had characteristic features. This patient's family required genetic advice and an explanation of the X-linked recessive transmission of the disorder. The advent of a gene probe to determine the carrier status will hopefully reduce the occurrence of this disease in the future.

173. This man has dermatitis herpetiformis; the picture shows a crop of itchy blisters in a typical position. The vesicles are ruptured by scratching, heal by crusting over and often leave pigmented scars. Also, there is often an associated gluten enteropathy. Skin biopsy shows that the blisters are subepidermal in situation and immunofluorescence shows the present of granular IgA deposits in the dermal papillae. Jejunal biopsy will confirm the presence of gluten enteropathy. The differential diagnosis of this blistering condition includes porphyria cutanea tardia and drug-associated allergy. The recommended treatment is with dapsone, and if there is proven gluten sensitivity a gluten-free diet should be recommended.

174. This picture shows marked wasting of the right thenar eminence and clinical examination of sensation showed impairment of sensation over the thumb and adjacent two and a half fingers, plus the radial half of the palm of the hand. This represents the distribution of the median nerve. The patient had realised that she could relieve the pain by elevation of the hand or gentle shaking of the hand in the air (flick test). The additional tests that should be done are:

(a) Tinel's test, which consists of tapping with a finger over the carpal tunnel. This produces paraesthesia in the hand and pain may travel up the arm.

(b) Phalen's test, which has the same basis as Tinel's test, but here the stimulus is flexion of the wrist for about one minute, producing paraesthesia in the hand.

(c) Application of an upper arm tourniquet results in sensory deficit.

The diagnosis should be confirmed with nerve conduction studies of the lower arm. Surgical decompression of the carpal tunnel is often required unless there is some obvious self-limiting or treatable disease, e.g. pregnancy or hypothyroidism. Steroid injection into the carpal tunnel has been used for symptomatic relief and may occasionally be curative.

175.   The x-ray appearances are those of renal rickets with characteristic changes in the epiphysis at the lower end of the radius; the epiphyseal cartilage is expanded and thickened and the distal ends of the shafts are widened, manifesting the typical "saucer" deformity. There is also delay in bone calcification. This boy had renal impairment that progressed to end-stage renal disease, and he is now on dialysis. In this type of patient one would expect to find a reduction of plasma calcium level, an increased plasma phosphate, increased alkaline phosphatase and low values for 1,25 hydroxy vitamin D_3.

176.   Clinical inspection of the patient shows that the pupils are of different size, and they are both regular. The right pupil reacts sluggishly to direct light and also to accommodation. This patient has the Holmes-Adie syndrome (myotonic pupil). It is of no pathological significance but may be associated with hypo- or areflexia. The site of the lesion is unknown and the disorder is commoner in women than in men. There are no medical consequences and the patient can be reassured.

177.   There is an increase in the bronchovascular markings, particularly at both bases, extending right out to the periphery of the lung fields, and the diaphragms are high. These are the typical features of early fibrosing alveolitis. The best clinical clue was the presence of numerous inspiratory crepitations, which were particularly marked at the end of inspiration and present bilaterally over the lower zones. Pulmonary function tests showed a restrictive ventilatory defect with a reduction in lung volume and a low carbon monoxide transfer factor. The measurement of the arterial oxygen level showed a low value, particularly at the end of exercise.

178.   This is the Ramsay Hunt syndrome, which results from herpes zoster affecting the geniculate ganglion of the VIIth nerve. The patients present with a VIIth nerve palsy on the same side and a herpetic rash with typical vesicles in the external auditory meatus, as shown here, and in the pharynx (small sensory branches of VII innervate both the external meatus and the pharynx). Treatment with acyclovir alters the natural history of the disease and results in more rapid recovery of nerve function. Most patients recover total function of the nerve.

179.   These are severe pressure sores, which have occurred in a 55-year-old man with multiple sclerosis. He has been bed-bound and incontinent for some years. Such sores inevitably become infected and the major complication is perforation into adjacent tissues with resulting osteomyelitis and septicaemia. Pressure sores of this type are extremely difficult to treat and it is important to emphasize that prevention is of great importance in patients at risk. These particular sores have been treated over several weeks and the infection and sloughing areas have been removed. The patient is being prepared for an attempt at skin grafting, but the outcome is difficult to predict, due to the underlying disease and the patient's incontinence.

180.   This x-ray of the cervical spine shows the advanced changes associated with ankylosing spondylitis. There is rigid ankylosis with calcification of the spinal ligament. In addition, the spine is severely demineralized and has lost its normal curvature. These changes have the appearance of bamboo spine, which is more commonly seen in the lumbar area. This patient had severe restriction of movement with limited mobility; he was unable to rotate his head and, as a result, had stopped driving. In addition, he had iritis with visual impairment and aortic valve disease, although this was not symptomatic. He subsequently tripped and fell while at home, and the violent movement was sufficient to fracture his C2 vertebra.

181. This is a typical lesion of contagious pustular dermatitis (orf), which is due to a pox virus infection of sheep and goats that usually affects the animals' lips. It is a common complication in those working with animals and it presents as a firm, painless, purple- coloured papule usually on the fingers and hands. The condition is self limiting and usually clears within four to eight weeks.

182. This is a carotid artery angiogram, showing a right posterior communicating artery aneurysm. The clinical presentation of the patient is characteristic of subarachnoid haemorrhage, in that she presented with sudden-onset severe headache, extreme vomiting and neck pain; no focal signs were present but she had neck stiffness and a positive straight leg raising test. The fundi were normal and did not show papilloedema or subhyaloid haemorrhages. CT scan carried out on the night of admission showed the characteristic appearances of blood in the subarachnoid space. A clip was applied to ablate the aneurysm in a subsequent surgical operation.

183. The abnormalities seen here are the colour of the toes, which are a deep blue-purple, especially in the nailbed (this is an extreme degree of cyanosis), and the drumstick appearance of the ends of the toes, which results from toe clubbing. In a lateral view it would be more apparent that the angle between the nail and the nailbed is filled in. There is also increased curvature of the nail and, with the amount of collagen laid down, the nail apppears to float on the nailbed when palpated. While there are many different causes of finger and toe clubbing, the presence of such severe cyanosis in a young person almost always represents some congenital abnormality of the great vessels, which results in cyanotic heart disease. Most common is Fallot's tetralogy, but in this patient the underlying abnormality was partial transposition of the great vessels.

184. This patient was seen in the cardiology clinic, having been admitted with a murmur that was diagnosed as mitral stenosis. This was confirmed by echocardiography. The appearance of the patient's cheeks was put down to "malar flush". However, in this case the distribution has more of a "butterfly" or "bat wing" appearance, with an area of erythema on the bridge of the nose. The possibility of concomitant lupus erythematosus was debated, while the other possibility was unrelated acne rosacea. The rash of acne rosacea, however, tends to be more blotchy, with papules and pustules and occasionally keratitis. It is particularly relevant that there were no other clinical features suggestive of lupus erythematosus. In particular, no joints or other areas of skin were involved, there were no nail changes or evidence of Raynaud's disease, and no purpura. The patient's erythrocyte sedimentation rate (ESR) was normal and a screen of auto-antibodies, including the DNA antibody test, were negative. The importance of malar flush as a sign of mitral stenosis has probably been grossly over-emphasized, and other causes, even a perfectly healthy but ruddy appearance, should always be considered.

185. This is an ultrasound of the gallbladder area, which is the optimal initial investigation for patients suspected of having gallstones. The advantages are that the procedure is non-invasive, cheap and easily repeatable. The examination shows a rather dilated gallbladder with an irregular stone clearly visible within it. Note also the acoustic shadow thrown by the stone, which is a typical and helpful feature of the investigation.

186. These changes in the nails are long standing. There is onycholysis, a yellow-brownish pigmentation, with pitting and ridging, and the nails are soft, friable and easily split. The underlying cause is chronic infection with *Candida albicans.* The patient has chronic mucocutaneous candidiasis, which normally begins in childhood and may be associated with autoimmune endocrine diorders including hypoadrenalism, hypothyroidism or diabetes mellitus. In adults the condition may be associated with the presence of a thymoma. *Candida* infection may involve most areas of the skin and mucos membranes, and it does not respond to conventional treatment. Lengthy, intensive treatment is required to eliminate this fungal nail infection.

187. There is gross atrophy of the muscles of the shoulder cuff; in particular, the deltoid has almost totally disappeared and the other upper arm muscles are extremely atrophic. There is gross disorganization of the shoulder joint (a Charcot joint); these changes were bilateral. The patient has syringomyelia, the symptoms and signs of which had been progressive during the preceding few years. Other possible causes include tertiary syphilis, diabetes mellitus, and a range of rare disorders associated with sensory neuropathy. However, in the shoulder, syringomyelia is the most likely cause.

188. This is a two-dimensional echocardiogram in the parasternal long-axis view. The main abnormality is gross dilatation of the proximal aorta (**AO**). There is also a linear echo within the aortic lumen, which could be an intimal flap. The appearances are strongly suggestive of a dissecting aneurysm of the ascending aorta.

189. This woman has a large thyroid nodule arising from the left lobe of the thyroid, the scar of a previous thyroidectomy and the features of hypothyroidism. In particular she has a puffy face and puffiness in the supraclavicular fossae, her hair is unkempt and she has lost the lateral third of her eyebrows. Examination showed the skin to be cold and dry, and she had bradycardia (60bpm). The clinical suspicion of hypothyroidism was confirmed by measuring T4 and TSH. It is important on clinical examination of such a thyroid nodule to determine whether it is asymmetrical, ascertain its consistency and whether there is associated lymphadenopathy, whether the nodule has increased rapidly in size, perhaps due to haemorrhage, whether there is any hoarseness and whether the nodule is attached to the skin or underlying tissue. It should be investigated using thyroid scanning or ultrasound. Following this a fine needle aspiration for cytology should be carried out. About 95 per cent of thyroid nodules are benign. It is important to find out what operation was carried out previously, how much of the thyroid was removed and what additional treatment was given. In particular, was the patient exposed to therapeutic doses of radioactive iodine?

190. This patient has a large gastric ulcer, in the base of which there is a small thrombosed vessel. This was the cause of the presenting symptomatology, which was haematemesis and melaena. It is important to examine the edges of gastric ulcers carefully; the upper edge of this ulcer is rolled, which points to malignancy. Multiple biopsies should be taken as near to this edge as possible. In the meantime, specific therapy should be given either with H_2

blockers or with a proton pump inhibitor such as omeprazole. If the biopsy shows no evidence of malignancy the patient should be re-endoscoped in three months to confirm that the ulcer is healing and, if necessary, biopsies should be repeated.

191. The major abnormalities in this x-ray are: the striking degree of pericardial calcification and the presence of a wire suture in the sternum. The patient has had surgery to remove much of his calcified pericardium, the wire suture representing the operative site. Note that the sternum is rather badly aligned at this point. The patient had presented with an insidious onset of heart failure, with distension of neck veins, peripheral oedema, ascites and hepatic congestion. He also had pulsus paradoxus. Chest x-ray showed pericardial calcification while ECG showed low-voltage QRS complexes and T-wave inversion. Echocardiography revealed the thickened pericardium. The diagnosis was constrictive pericarditis, associated with pericardial calcification. The aetiology of this condition in individual patients is often not clear; it is known to follow tuberculous pericarditis (still probably the commonest cause worldwide), but it may also follow episodes of viral or bacterial infection or rheumatic fever. Pericardectomy resulted in a dramatic response, with loss of the features of heart failure.

192. This woman has a very prominent corneal arcus, which is probably significant at this age and prompts investigation of her lipid profile. The second abnormality is in her pupil, which is extremely small and irregular, and was not responsive to light directly or consensually, although it did react to accommodation. Both eyes were similarly affected. The Argyll Robertson pupil as shown here is a feature of tertiary neurosyphilis, and this patient had other evidence of general paralysis of the insane, with progressive dementia and the reflexes of a generalized upper motor neurone lesion, i.e. risk tendon jerks and extensor plantar responses. This abnormality has become extraordinarily rare in Western society due to the fall in the number of cases of teritiary syphilis, but similar pupil abnormality may occasionally be seen in diabetes mellitus.

193. The appearances here are those of late retinitis pigmentosa. There is attenuation of the retinal arteries, pallor of the optic disc and large amounts of typical "bone corpuscle" pigmentation, which has been progressively produced by retinal cells. The disease results from the metabolic disturbance of the photoreceptor and retinal pigment epithelial cells, whose function it is to phagocytose photochemical pigments.

About 50 per cent of patients have a family history of the disease, which may be inherited an X-linked, dominant or recessive trait. In this instance the patient had been adopted so no gene probe studies could be carried out.

As yet there is no treatment.

194. This is the typical cutaneous lesion of anthrax (often called a "malignant pustule"), which had started as a small pimple 3 days prior to this picture, and grew rapidly. The centre of the lesion ulcerated and the base of the ulcer was covered with this firmly adherent black scab.

Veterinary surgeons are particularly at risk from this infection, while other groups include farmers, butchers, abbatoir workers and anyone who works with animal products, perhaps in a tannery or with bone meal. This patient habitually carried animal hides by slinging them around his neck.

The diagnosis may be made by direct Gram staining of a scraping form the lesion, which demonstrates Gram-positive rods.

Penicillin by intramuscular injection remains the antibiotic of choice. Vaccination is available for workers at high risk.

195. This patient has perioral dermatitis. Severe perioral dermatitis is most likely to be caused by the inappropriate use (prescription or self-medication) of topical steroids for facial skin disorders. In this case, topical corticosteroids had been used, and a lip-licking habit may have exacerbated the condition

Potent topical steroids should never be used on the face, and facial eczema should never be treated with anything stronger than the lowest-strength hydrocortisone.

196. The major abnormality in the first film is a large nodular lesion in the left upper zone. The nodule contains a fluid level, so it is cavitating. The most likely diagnosis is lung cancer, although cavitating nodules may also occur in other conditions including Wegener's granulomatosis and rheumatoid arthritis. The second film shows consolidation of the left upper lobe and paratracheal lymph node enlargement. The patient had lung cancer, which progressed to obstruct the left upper lobe boundaries, despite radiotherapy in the intervening period.

197. There is marked frontal baldness, bilateral ptosis, facial weakness and atrophy of the sternomastoids, masseters and temporalis muscles. These are the visible features of dystrophia myotonica. There were no cataracts present but the patinet had gonadal atrophy. ECG and ultrasound of his heart showed no evidence of cardiomyopathy.

The cause of the disease is a gene defect associated with chromosome 19. There is a useful surrogate marker for the complement C3 locus, which is adjacent and can be used for linkage analysis in family studies.

There is no specific treatment. Development of cataracts is common and patients should be reviewed for this reason.

198. This ia a contrast-enhanced coronal CT scan of the head, showing the region of the pituitary fossa. A pituitary tumour is present, which extends above the level of the normal pituitary fossa.

The tumour is encroaching on the left optic radiation, which can be seen immediately above and to the right of the tumour in the image. Visual field defects are likely to result from compression of the optic radiation, chiasma or nerves.

The tumour was a prolactinoma, and the patient a 30-year-old woman who presented with infertility.

199. The abnormality illustrated is ectopic calcification in the lateral and nasal margins of the cornea. This is band keratopathy and the patient has hyperparathyroidism. The diagnosis was confirmed by an elevated plasma calcium and a low phosphate level. There was elevation of alkaline phosphatase and measurement of the parathormone level was diagnostic. Subperiosteal erosions are usually seen in bone x-ray in patients with this severity and duration of disease. There may also occasionally be bone cysts, which are best seen in the hands and skull. Stone formation is one of the common complications, due to deposition of calcium salts. Ectopic calcification may occur in a variety of tissues including the skin, kidney and cornea. Treatment of the hyperparathyroidism is surgical. Localization of the production of parathormone by selective venous sampling is followed by surgical resection.

200.   This woman has gross hypertrichosis, the cause of which is most to be diazoxide, a vasodilator drug that is used in severe hypertension, and also in the treatment of hypoglycaemia, especially where there is an inoperable insulinoma. Diazoxide is now used topically as a treatment for baldness.

INDEX

INDEX